CLINIQUE SCIENCE

WEIGHT LOSS

A simple method for losing weight rapidly and completely,
while improving your health, and reducing your risk of
developing heart disease, cancer, and a variety of other diseases

Dr. George M. Ekema

With special contributions from Dr. Marjet Heitzer

Edited by Marjet Heitzer

Medlife Publishing, Inc.

Published by Medlife Publishing, Inc.

Printed in the United States of America

ISBN 978-0–9768150-2-0

To my beloved father

Hon W. B. Ekema

(Mola Mbamba)

"...And though I have the gift of prophecy, and understand all mysteries and all knowledge, and though I have all faith, so that I could remove mountains, but have not love, I am nothing. And though I bestow all my goods to feed the poor, and though I give my body to be burned, but have not love, it profits me nothing. Love suffers long and is kind; love does not envy; love does not parade itself, is not puffed up; does not behave rudely, does not seek its own, is not provoked, thinks no evil; does not rejoice in iniquity, but rejoices in the truth; bears all things, believes all things, hopes all things, endures all things. Love never fails."
  - The Apostle Paul to the Corinthians - I.13.2-8.

You lived it Daddy!

Acknowledgments

Special thanks to Dr. Marjet Heitzer for her invaluable research on weight loss and the insightful articles thereof that are included in this book. Also for her editorial work on this book and her continuous editorial work on Trimming America (www.trimmingamerica.com).

I would also like to give special thanks to my family for their love, understanding and support – particularly for the patience that allowed me to complete this work.

To the hundreds of scientists (cited) who made this work possible – thank you.

Contents

------Chapter Two------

Medicinal foods and health management foods

------Chapter Four------

The plateau-proof diet

------Chapter Five------

The plateau-proof diet cardio – A healthier heart version of the plateau-proof diet

------Chapter Six------

Ready, Set, Go!!!

Introduction

Important warning: Please do not (under any circumstance) use this book or follow any of the information it contains without first consulting with your primary health care provider or other qualified clinician.

The clinique science weight loss system is a simple method of eating and living that will lead to a rapid and complete weight loss. Along with weight loss, the system targets health and wellness, holding strongly to the fact that a healthy body will lose weight faster than an unhealthy one. A healthier body is also more likely to maintain leanness following weight loss. The core of the system consists of medicinal foods and the plateau-proof diet (or the plateau-proof diet cardio).

Among the medicinal foods are herbs and spices that cause weight loss, but also medicinal foods for a broad range of diseases. Some of these foods may treat or cure health conditions while others may prevent health conditions from developing.

The plateau-proof diet (or the plateau-proof diet cardio) is a well-structured 2 rotation diet designed to eliminate or minimize the dreaded weight loss plateau and affect a complete weight loss. The diet is also designed to prevent or minimize weight gain following complete weight loss.

How to use the clinique science weight loss system

Step 1 – Your safety
The first step in using the clinique weight loss system is consulting with your primary health care provider (PCP) or other

qualified clinician. When cleared by your PCP or other clinician to use the system, enter the information in the table below. This information will help guide your priorities as you use the system. Recording this information also allows you to compare and track the progress of your health and weight loss. Repeat this screening every six months or as recommended by your PCP or other clinician. Use the forms in Appendix I to record the results.

Date_____

Screen	Your levels	Desirable levels
Total cholesterol		under 200 mg/dl
HDL cholesterol		45 mg/dl or higher
LDL cholesterol		100 mg/dl or lower
Triglycerides		under 150 mg/dl
Glucose		70-99 mg/dl fasting and below 140 mg/dl non-fasting
Blood pressure		systolic under 120 diastolic under 80
Body Mass Index (BMI)		between 18.5 and 25

Once you have received clearance from your PCP, you may proceed with the clinique science weight loss system. If your results indicate that you have type II diabetes, it is recommended that you use the type II diabetes edition of the clinique science weight loss system. Also, if the results of your screening indicate that you have high blood pressure, please use the hypertension edition of the clinique science weight loss system. If your total cholesterol level, LDL cholesterol level or triglyceride level is higher than normal and your blood pressure and glucose levels are normal use this edition of the clinique science weight loss and follow the plateau-proof diet cardio rather than the plateau-proof diet. If all your screening parameters are normal except for your BMI, use this edition of the clinique science weight loss with either the plateau-proof diet or the plateau-proof diet cardio.

Step 2 – the medicinal foods
Get your weight loss medicinal foods. Also get preventive and/or curative medicinal foods for the conditions that concern you. Make oil infusions or herbal teas of the medicinal foods where applicable (See Chapter 2).

Step 3 – the plateau-proof diet or the plateau-proof diet cardio
Start the plateau-proof diet or the plateau-proof diet cardio following the directions as described in chapters 4 and 5.
Use the oil infusions of medicinal foods (from step 2) to spice and flavor your foods as you normally would with salt and pepper or table condiments. Substitute soft drinks and other drinks that do not comply with the diet with the drinks that actively cause weight loss as described later in this book.

Step 4 – of mind and muscles

Most people with normal health screening parameters (step 1) are going to lose weight rapidly on the clinique science weight loss system without exercising. If you have elevated levels of glucose or triglycerides, it may be necessary for you to engage in very moderate exercise to accelerate your weight loss. The exercise is not intended to burn fat or burn calories, so do not engage in very strenuous exercise. Rather, the exercise is intended to complement the medicinal foods that make muscle cells improve their uptake and utilization of glucose and fat from the blood – both of which are compromised in most obese individuals and those with type II diabetes. Soon after starting the clinique science weight loss system, the muscle cells will be able to uptake and utilize glucose and fat with significantly increased efficiency – as you will see from subsequent health screening results. Choose exercises that will stimulate the larger muscles that form the bulk of your body – e.g. walking (or jogging), pushups, sit-ups, and leg squats. You will derive more benefit from exercising if you do not overdo it.

Here is an example of a good exercise regimen:

Monday – Walk (jog) 1 – 1.5 miles, doing half the distance at a brisk pace. Ideally you should alternate between a brisk pace and a leisurely pace in 0.1 mile intervals.

Wednesday – Pushups (partial or complete depending on your strength). Do 5 – 10 pushups or until you feel slight pain in arm or shoulder. Repeat 5 times, getting adequate rest between each set.

Friday – Sit-ups (partial or complete depending on your strength). Do 5 – 10 sit-ups or until you feel slight pain in belly or waist. Repeat 5 times, getting adequate rest between each set.

Saturday – Walk (jog) 1 – 1.5 miles, doing half the distance at a brisk pace. Ideally you should alternate between a brisk pace and a leisurely pace in 0.1 mile intervals.

As you can see, it is unnecessary to have a gym membership or "break sweat" to enjoy the benefits of exercise on the clinique science weight loss.

Of the mind
Everyone on the clinique science weight loss system, any other weight loss system, or any endeavor in life for that matter, could facilitate their journey and possibly improve their results by thinking positively. Essentially, it is important that you have a deep belief in yourself. Your belief (in yourself) should be strong enough to allow you to mentally or spiritually create an image of yourself as you desire to be (physically) when your weight loss is complete. Adopt the mental part of this image immediately – now visualizing yourself as temporarily trapped in the wrong body. It is going to be an interesting and challenging journey escaping from this body, but you are up to the task. You have facilitated your task and made it more fun by choosing this great tool – the clinique science weight loss system.

Important warning
Please do not (under any circumstance) use this book or follow any of the information it contains without first consulting with your primary health care provider or other qualified clinician.

Chapter One

Weight loss facts and fiction

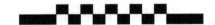

A few years ago while browsing weight loss products online, I found a company that sold sunglasses for weight loss. Hopefully you didn't buy one of these, but don't feel terrible if you did – you probably were not the only one. I continued browsing products and it didn't take long for me to realize that the weight loss market was a dumping ground for fictitious and silly gadgets from unscrupulous people trying to make a quick buck. I came across supplements and potions so ridiculous that I had to buy a few to test in my lab. Of course I wasn't testing them for efficacy on weight loss, since there was zero scientific backing for their weight loss claims. I simply wanted to know what was contained (actually) in these capsules, tablets, etc. In lab, I was unable to test some of the tablets because they couldn't dissolve in water or any other solvent for that matter. I heated water to boiling and these things still did not dissolve. I added strong acid and base – still did not dissolve. Testing complete - the conclusion is that these pills will fall in the toilet hours after they are eaten, and be identical to those still in the bottle. The effect on weight loss will be similar to swallowing glass buttons or marbles. Since you most likely do not have a lab or other means to test weight loss products and weight loss claims, I decided that I was going to start this book by catching you up with weight loss facts and fiction. Actually, I didn't just decide, I decided after convincing Dr. Marjet Heitzer to compile, research and write on the most important and vital weight loss and related (health) topics. The short passages you are about to read below are from Dr. Heitzer. I have learned quite a bit from them, and I hope you will too. I will be commenting in small boxes like the one below along the way.

> *The more you know about weight loss and its related health issues, the easier it will be for you to lose weight and keep it off, especially because you will be able to improvise – a very important but often overlooked aspect of a successful weight loss. Equally as important, you will eliminate the guesswork and avoid being a victim of weight loss myths.*

Does eating after 8:00 p.m. induce more weight gain?

The short answer to this question is- NO. Although this myth has been perpetuated for many years, it is a myth nonetheless. Because individuals are more likely to be sedentary (less active) later in the day, the myth states that you won't burn off the food eaten late at night. Because late night meals and snacks aren't immediately burned off, it is stored, hence weight gain.

In this article, we will find out that consuming a meal or snack late in the evening has no additional consequences as eating a meal or snack in the morning in reference to weight gain. Rather, it is the total amount of food as well as the combination of macronutrients (protein, carbohydrate, or fat) consumed during a 24 hour period which is more important.

So, what was the basis of this myth? After a great deal of searching, we discovered one very small study that included only 10 slightly to moderately obese women eating a controlled diet (provided by the study investigators). The authors of this study determined that there was a slight enhancement in weight loss when individuals consumed higher daily energy in the morning (breakfast and lunch) as opposed to the evening (dinner and evening snack)[8]. In the first 6 weeks, the time of day in which most of the food was consumed did not matter. However, in the following 6 weeks, the investigators observed that women, who consumed most of their food energy in the morning hours, lost slightly more weight (8.6 and 7.2 lbs., respectively) than women who consumed more food in the evening. However, women that had the evening meal schedule lost less fat-free (or lean) mass, indicating that they had a greater loss of body fat percentage. It should be restated that the results indicated only a slight benefit from consuming most of their food in the morning. Also, because the number of participants in this study as well as the length of the study was very small, it is difficult to determine if this trend would continue.

Although meal time does not directly affect weight gain, people that eat breakfast are relatively less prone to obesity. There is some evidence that people who consume more food in the morning hours tend to consume less total food[9]. A study by deCastro *et al.* observed 375 men and 492 women eating *ad libitum* (at their own discretion) using a diet journal system[9]. They found that consuming food in the morning may provide more satiety (the feeling of fullness) as compared to eating food later in the day. This may be why meal sizes tend to increase and between meal intervals decrease as the day progresses, resulting in ingestion of approximately 150% more food energy in the evening as compared to the morning. So, people who tend to consume more food in the evening hours were inclined to consume more total food. It may be that eating breakfast and a larger lunch influences an individual's feeling of hunger, thereby influencing the amount of total food consumed in a day.

Obese people tend to consume more food than normal sized people and most of that food is eaten in the evening[10]. Although consuming food in the evening doesn't affect weight gain directly, if a person skips breakfast and consumes most of their food in the evening, they generally eat more, leading to increased weight gain. Alternatively, people who eat breakfast tend to consume less food totally throughout the day.

It should be noted that this portion is concerned with moderate evening meal and snack consumption and not excessive evening eating as in night eating syndrome (NES). NES is characterized by morning anorexia, evening hyperphagia (enormous overeating), as well as insomnia[11]. Individuals suffering from NES are fully awake and conscious during these episodes. Most people with NES consume more that 50% of their daily caloric intake after their last evening meal in the form of evening snack[12]. Although NES is often associated with obesity, it can be present in non-obese individuals[13]. Finally, NES is also associated with depression. If you think you may be suffering from NES, it is important to immediately contact your primary care physician to discuss relevant treatment options.

Being a night person I am glad to know that eating late does not lead to weight gain. I know that we (night eaters) tend to eat a little more than the early risers, so I tend to control my portions. Nothing too drastic, essentially making sure that the signal of fullness is not the stretching of my abdomen. Several smaller portions of food eaten over time tend to be better than one large portion for weight loss.

Also, make sure that you include your medicinal foods (see the next chapter) with every meal, especially the weight loss herbs and/or spices and the spices that regulate the metabolism of sugar and fat.

Morning people have even more of an advantage eating these medicinal foods with breakfast. Please include my potent herbal weight loss tea (I will discuss this tea a little later) with breakfast and other meals.

A Hearty Buzz from Alcohol

In recent years, moderate consumption of alcohol, particularly red wine, has been associated with various health benefits including lowering the risk of coronary heart disease (CHD, atherosclerosis), ischemic stroke (interrupted blood flow to the brain due to a blood clot or bursting of a blood vessel) and cerebral thrombosis (blood clot in the brain). For example, light to moderate drinkers have less risk of developing CHD than abstainers[14]. However, heavy drinking actually raises a person's risk of developing CHD. This article will examine scientific evidence associated with alcohol consumption and CHD. However, this article is by no means promoting increased alcohol consumption in order to attain cardioprotection. Alcoholism is associated with many more health problems such as liver cirrhosis, cancer, neurological diseases as well as heart complications like alcoholic cardiomyopathy (weakening of the heart muscle seen in some chronic alcoholics) and high blood pressure. Individuals should discuss alcohol consumption with their physician.

Part of the epidemiological evidence associated with the benefits of alcohol consumption, particularly red wine, comes from the French Paradox[15]. Despite the high amounts of saturated fat in their diet, the French have a relatively low incidence of CHD. Comparing the eating and drinking habits of European countries that have low rates of CHD resulted in a common factor: consumption of more red wine as compared to other countries. This led to the question: Could red wine consumption lead to heart health benefits?

In the Copenhagen City Heart Study, 13,285 men and women

were observed for twelve years[16]. Individuals, who drank wine, had 50% less CHD. In this study, beer and spirit drinkers had no reduction in CHD. However, another similar study indicated that moderate beer consumption decreased the risk of CHD by 22%[17].

So what is CHD? Atherosclerosis is the accumulation of fatty plaques in blood vessels, leading to decreased blood flow to the heart. One of the initial steps in the progression of atherosclerosis is the inability of the blood vessels to relax or vasodilate. Smoking, hypertension (high blood pressure), high cholesterol, and diabetes are just a few complications that may be responsible for reduced vasodilation. Proliferation and migration of smooth muscle cells underneath the endothelium (cells lining the blood vessels) results in decreased blood vessel relaxation and a thickening of the blood vessel wall. In the end, the plaque ruptures and leads to either a heart attack or stroke.

In laboratory studies, alcohol improves endothelial cell (the cells that line blood vessels) function and inhibits vascular smooth muscle cell proliferation and migration, resulting in more relaxed blood vessels[18]. Furthermore, red wine reduced the production of endothelin-1, a protein involved in blood vessel vasoconstriction[19]. Finally, alcohol consumption leads to decreased LDL (bad cholesterol) oxidation, increased HDL (good cholesterol) concentrations, and decreased platelet aggregation, resulting in a better blood lipid profile and less plaque formation[18]. Taken together, alcohol itself improves vascular function, resulting in reduced risk of developing CHD.

So, why does wine, especially red wine, have additional health benefits as opposed to beer or spirits? Studies using dealcolized red wine showed that some of the cardioprotective characteristics of red wine are independent of the alcohol. Along with alcohol, red and white wine are composed of many other chemicals from the grape, including polyphenols that act as antioxidants. However, red wine typically has more antioxidant polyphenols than white wine. Plant polyphenols are responsible for the color of the grape. Red wine has a variety of polyphenols including resveratrol (stilbene) and flavinoids. The antioxidant function of red wine flavinoids decreases LDL (bad cholesterol) oxidation[20]. Because oxidized LDL reduces blood vessel relaxation, it is a crucial step leading to heart disease. Along with reducing oxidized LDL concentrations, polyphenols may also reduce cholesterol absorption in the gut, leading to decreased serum cholesterol concentrations. Finally, grape polyphenols decrease plasma triglyceride concentrations by 39%[21]. All of these changes may result in suppression of atherosclerosis, thus reduced risk of developing CHD.

What is moderate and heavy consumption of alcohol? Moderate consumption of alcoholic beverages (1-2 drinks/day) 3 to 4 days per week results in a 30% reduction in risk of developing CHD and a 20% reduction in the risk of developing ischemic stroke. Each drink consists of 1.5 ounces of liquor, 5 ounces of wine, or 12 ounces of beer. However, heavy drinking as well as binge or weekend drinking (5+ drinks for women and 9+ drinks for men) are not associated with any cardioprotective effects. In fact, heavy and binge drinkers had a higher risk of developing CHD as compared to abstainers.

Do only healthy individuals benefit from moderate alcohol consumption? Healthy individuals along with patients with a history of heart attack or diabetes all may benefit from moderate drinking. Men with a history of ischemic heart disease had an increase in blood vessel size after ingestion of both red and white wine[22]. Furthermore, in a model of insulin resistance, insulin resistant rats benefited from the consumption of alcohol, red wine polyphenols, or both[23]. In this model of insulin resistance, rats are fed a high fructose diet that leads to metabolic syndrome followed by glucose intolerance, visceral obesity, hypertension, insulin resistance, and dyslipidemia. Drinking alcohol or red wine polyphenols led to increased insulin sensitivity, in turn resulting in lower blood glucose and normal blood pressure. Rats that consumed alcohol alone had decreased insulin resistance.

With the many options for cardioprotection listed in the medicinal foods portion of this book, it is unnecessary to start drinking alcohol just to enjoy its benefits. Also, if alcohol is currently part of your diet, your risk of developing CHD may be significantly lowered by consuming moderate levels of the right kind of alcohol(s). Excessive consumption of alcohol may increase your risk for developing heart disease and other diseases.

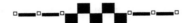

A more recent study showed some cardiovascular health benefits even to weekend warriors. Binge drinking a couple of nights a week though is certainly NOT the way to go. Remember that alcohol is an energy rich fuel for the body, and while very moderate (see daily drink quantity recommendations below) consumption may help you lose weight and improve your cardiovascular health, amounts over 'very moderate' may lead to additional weight gain and other health complications.

Recommended beverage consumption pattern:
- **Water 50 oz or more**
- **Tea/Coffee 28 oz**
- **Fat-free milk 16 oz**
- **No calorie sweetened beverage 0-16 oz**
- **Caloric beverages with nutrients (alcohol/some fruit juices) 0-16 oz**

Land a punch on fat – Go Nuts!

Nuts are an excellent source of protein as well as fiber, vitamin E, and omega-3 fatty acids. Although nuts are an energy rich food, composed of 45-75% fat depending on the type of nut, that fat is largely unsaturated. Along with the benefits of higher fiber, vitamin E, and omega-3 fatty acid consumption, nuts provide other health benefits such as increasing insulin sensitivity, endothelial cell (the cells that line blood vessels) function, and decreasing blood lipid (cholesterol) levels, thereby decreasing the risk of coronary heart disease (CHD).

Recent studies suggest that consumption of nuts, particularly almonds, peanuts, pecan nuts, and walnuts may benefit the heart, and actively contribute to weight loss. Particularly, eating 4-5 servings (50-100 grams/day) each week lowers blood lipid levels and LDL (bad cholesterol) within a few short weeks when it is substituted for traditional, highly saturated fats[24]. Furthermore, 1 ounce of nuts per day decreases the risk of fatal coronary heart disease by 45% when they are substituted for saturated fat and 30% when substituted for carbohydrates[25]. The lipid lowering affects of nuts were seen in both lean and obese individuals, with and without hypercholesterolemia, indicating that consumption of nuts may decrease cholesterol levels in individuals with preexisting high cholesterol[26]. It should be noted here that not all nuts reduced cholesterol levels. Increased consumption of macadamia nuts as well as hazelnuts did not alter cholesterol levels, indicating that the health benefits from eating nuts may not be gained if those nuts are selected.

There is epidemiological (studies involving the distribution of health-related issues within certain populations) evidence that areas such as the Mediterranean region that consume a diet rich in nuts have a lower proportion of sudden cardiac death. Furthermore, there is an inverse relationship between nut consumption and sudden cardiac death as well as obesity, meaning that a person that consumes more nuts is less likely to die from CHD or to be obese. Finally, nut consumption is inversely associated with the risk of development of type II diabetes, presumably because individuals who consume nuts on a regular basis are less likely to be obese[27].

How do nuts decrease the risk of coronary heart disease? First, nuts are composed mainly of monounsaturated fats, and substitution of foods containing saturated fat with unsaturated fat will improve blood lipid levels, thereby decreasing the risk of heart disease. Additionally, nuts are a great source of other heart healthy items, such as vitamin E, fiber, magnesium, potassium and arginine.

Vitamin E has antioxidant properties, making it a great vitamin in the fight against heart disease. In fact, Vitamin E is one of the most abundant naturally occurring antioxidants found in foods. Antioxidants protect against oxidative damage, a phenomenon that occurs in many diseases including heart disease and cancer[28]. Vitamin E inhibits the oxidation of LDL (bad cholesterol). Oxidation of LDL is one of the initial steps that occur during atherosclerosis, leading to endothelial cell damage as well as narrowing of blood vessels. Because nuts contain high amounts of the antioxidant vitamin E, it is thought that this may be one of many ways which they help lower your risk of CHD.

Omega-3 fatty acids are also found in nuts and have anti-atherogenic properties. Omega-3 fatty acids inhibit platelet aggregation (clot formation). Furthermore, omega-3 fatty acids improve endothelial function, protecting endothelial cells from damage[25]. Endothelial dysfunction occurs early in the progression of atherosclerosis (narrowing or hardening of the arteries). Studies have also reported an inverse relationship between fish oils that contain high amounts of omega-3 fatty acids and mortality from coronary heart disease[29].

Fiber has also been shown to have beneficial health benefits[30]. Fiber lowers blood cholesterol as well as decreasing hypertension (high blood pressure). Because most nuts are high in fiber, it is considered one of the many ways in which nut consumption leads to reduced risk of CHD. So, a combination of lowering blood cholesterol levels as well as improving endothelial function culminates in improved heart health with the consumption of nuts.

Several studies have addressed the question: Does increased nut consumption lead to weight gain? Although the beneficial effects of nuts on CHD have been well recognized, given the obesity epidemic in the United States physicians were concerned about possible weight gain induced by nut consumption because nuts are so high in fat - although it is the good, unsaturated fat. The resounding answer is No, nuts do not increase body mass index [(BMI) a means of measuring obesity]. In fact, there was an inverse relationship between nut consumption and BMI, indicating that a person eating nuts is less likely to be overweight[31]. In the above mentioned studies, there was no significant change in weight after increasing nut consumption. In fact, there was a small tendency towards weight loss while on the nut diet and females with the highest BMI actually lost weight[31]. Foods which are high in protein and unsaturated fat, such as nuts, may increase resting energy expenditure by increasing diet-induced thermogenesis. Furthermore, high fiber and protein foods tend to enhance satiety, or the feeling of being full.

Nuts whether used as food replacement or snacks are an excellent food choice for individuals who want to lose weight. Go nuts!

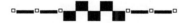

I have always known that nuts rule, but I have one major problem with them – they are too expensive. Of the four most beneficial nuts, three (almonds, pecan nuts and walnuts) are a treat for me. I certainly can't afford to snack on those regularly. Thank goodness peanuts are not as pricey. For that reason I have bonded with peanuts, eating at least a handful or two each day.

This is what is going on in my head as the nuts are making their way to my belly:
These tiny nuts are going to get into my belly then into my blood. They are going to instruct the cells of my muscles and organs to increase the amounts of glucose and fat that they absorb from my blood. More importantly they are going to instruct the cells of my muscles and organs to increase the metabolism of glucose and fat. If there is less glucose and fat in my blood something has to give, else my cells will starve. That is where the love handles come in. The fat cells in my love handles will have to dump their fat content into my blood. The nuts will again instruct the cells of my muscles and organs to pick up the fat from my blood and burn it. I am keeping this up until the nuts squeeze the fat dry out of my love handles.
***Of course you don't have to consciously think about it or meditate like I do, but I guarantee you that it helps to get the mind involved in weight loss. The power of positive thinking is amazing, and the constant visualization of goals and desired outcomes is the key. Your mind is a powerful thing; include it in your weight loss journey.
Go nuts!

The Holidays and Weight Loss Dieting – Still Oxymoronic to you?

Although the holidays are a time of celebration as well as reflection, they also represent a veritable dieting nightmare. Almost as a rule, each holiday party contains a wealth of food items deemed untouchable to most dieters. It is no mistake that following the revelries of holiday binges come the all-forgiving New Year's resolutions, which most likely include some of the characteristics such as overeating displayed during the previous weeks. This article will discuss some facts concerning weight loss maintenance during the holidays as well as some helpful hints to get you through them.

The average person gains approximately 1.1 pounds (0.5 kg) during the holiday season[32]. Furthermore, people of all sizes gain weight in December and January. Specifically, obese and normal-sized individuals gain 1.32 pounds (0.6 kg) and 0.88 pounds (0.4 kg), respectively[33]. Although gaining 1.1 pounds may seem like no big deal, for a person trying to lose weight, gaining instead of losing weight is devastating and may threaten their desire to continue dieting.

So, why do we gain weight during the holidays? As you can probably imagine, the reasons behind holiday weight gain are subjective, varying from person to person, as well as complex, possibly involving multiple factors such as financial and family stress along with increased social interactions surrounding foods (i.e. holiday parties). Although occasional binge episodes during the holiday seasons may seem harmless, there is evidence that people suffering from periodic overeating are less likely to continue a dieting regimen[34]. Furthermore, people, who occasionally overeat, are more likely to have a harder time controlling their weight.

There is some evidence that self-monitoring, the systematic observation or recording of target behaviors, may assist people during the holiday, helping individuals to stay focused on their diet[35]. In a study conducted by Baker *et al.*, participants that self-monitored, writing down their total food intake daily as well as the time the food was consumed and their weight each week, continued to lose weight during the holiday season[35]. However, the control group, participants that didn't self-monitor, gained 500% more weight over the holiday. Perhaps, self-monitoring serves as a checkpoint between putting a food item on your plate and into your mouth. Even outside of the holiday season, individuals that self-monitor, lost 64% more weight and continued with their diet as compared to participants that didn't self-monitor[36].

Perhaps self-monitoring provides some dieting consistency throughout the year. A recent study of the National Weight Control Registry, composed of people who lost significant amounts of weight and maintained their weight for 1 year, asked the question: Does consistency in dieting matter in weight loss maintenance? The answer was yes, people who maintained the same diet over weekdays, weekends, and holidays were 1½ times more likely to maintain their weight as compared to people that dieted strictly on the weekdays and non-holidays[37]. So, staying consistent throughout the holiday season as well as self-monitoring can help you get through the upcoming season, losing weight instead of gaining it.

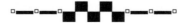

Soy – What's up?

In 1999, the FDA issued a statement which gave manufacturers permission to label products with high soy content as foods that may help lower the risk of heart disease. As a result, an explosion of soy-related products has hit U.S. grocery and drug stores in recent years. With the increased availability of soy-based food and supplements, comes a laundry list of ailments that can be alleviated with the convenient consumption of these products, including reducing the risk of breast cancer to an effective alternative to estrogen replacement therapy during menopause. While reading through the available literature on the benefits of soy consumption, I couldn't ignore the minor percentage of articles that pose a cautionary opinion on the health benefits of soy-related products. The details of those articles as well as the differences in soy-related foods and supplements to your health will be discussed.

The FDA recently published a statement indicating that foods containing soy protein along with a diet low in saturated fats and cholesterol may reduce the risk of coronary heart disease by lowering blood cholesterol levels. Over the years, significant amounts of research indicate that consumption of soy proteins reduces blood lipid levels, lowering LDL (bad cholesterol) levels. However, the question of how soy proteins lower cholesterol levels is still unanswered. In an attempt to add more soy-based foods into their diet, individuals replace animal-based foods, which are typically high in saturated fats, with soy-based foods. Lowering the consumption of animal-based foods alone lowers cholesterol, which combined with consumption of cholesterol-lowering soy proteins may reduce the risk of heart disease.

Along with the benefits of lowering cholesterol lipids, soy consumption has been associated with improving menopausal symptoms, reducing post-menopausal bone loss, as well as reducing the risk of hormone-related cancers, such as breast and prostate cancer[38]. These health benefits are most likely derived in part from the phytoestrogens (isoflavones) found in soy. The two major isoflavones found in soy are genistin/genistein and daidzin/diadzein.

Phytoestrogens possess estrogen-like properties, which is the basis for their use for post-menopausal symptoms and bone loss. During menopause, estrogen levels drop, leading to the onset of menopausal symptoms such as hot flashes, night sweats, vaginal dryness, and bone loss. Replacing the lost estrogen using hormone replacement therapy has been a traditional therapy used to alleviate the symptoms associated with menopause. The initial benefits from soy consumption on bone health were determined by epidemiological data that suggested that Asian women, whose diets are rich in soy-based foods, have a lower hip fracture rate as compared to their Western counterparts[39]. To this end, consumption of soy has recently been used as an alternative to estrogen replacement therapy for the management of menopausal symptoms. However, the emergence of soy supplements has led to increased concern associated with the safety of these supplements and possible risks.

Any food is composed of a complex ratio of macronutrients (carbs, fat, and protein) as well as vitamins, minerals, and other components. Soy-based foods are no exception. Most whole soy foods contain fiber, B vitamins, calcium, and omega-3 fatty acids as well as a myriad of other chemical components such as isoflavones. In many cases the benefits associated with the consumption of any food is linked to not just one individual isolate of that food, but a specific combination of components. So, isolation and purification of individual compounds within a food for use as a supplement does not always lead to the initial benefits of consumption of the whole food and should be approached with caution. In some cases, supplements actually raise the concentration of certain chemicals to toxic levels, thereby inducing health problems, not preventing them. This is the case for soy concentrates or isolates, isoflavone mixes and supplements. Some of the risks associated with soy consumption include increased risk of developing breast cancer, reduced cognitive function, and reproductive problems[40]. It should be noted here that most of the benefits associated with soy consumption come from consumption of whole soy foods and not supplements.   Furthermore, the FDA announcement includes soy foods made from the whole soybean and not supplements.

So, what are some examples of whole soy-based foods? Soy-based foods can be produced using all parts of the soy bean. For example, whole roasted or fermented soybeans themselves can be eaten. Alternatively, parts of the soy bean such as the hull or outer covering can be used to produce soy fiber.

No matter which soy-based foods you introduce into your diet, it is important that when substituting soy foods for dairy products such as milk, yogurt, or cheese, you choose soy foods which are calcium fortified. Because dairy foods are an important source of dietary calcium, calcium fortified soy products should be substituted for dairy products.

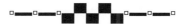

Soy beans and most soy products are disgusting to me. Several years ago when I decided to put my obligatory carnivore days behind me, I settled for tofu as a new non-animal protein source. I had tofu once or twice (when I could work up the courage) a week and those were some disgusting meals. It wasn't until I found the good (brown and hard) tofu in a Chinese store that I rescued myself from some serious nastiness. I still eat tofu once or twice a week and although I don't enjoy it as much as salmon or chicken meals, I could frankly include the word yummy in its description.

The point I am trying to make is that although most soy products are disgusting to me, I am able to enjoy the benefits of soy in the narrow margin of hard brown tofu that I have actually grown to like. I am certain that I am not the only one who finds soy products disgusting. If you too have problems with soy products, I suggest that you stay away from the soy products in your local grocery store. Go to an Asian store and explore – you may be pleasantly surprised.

Weight loss from Citrus?

Does drinking a small quantity of citrus juice in the morning jumpstart your metabolism?

The simple answer is NO. Although the basis of this dieting myth is elusive at best, it is possible that its creator heard about the Ephedra substitute, synephrine, found in the outer peel of *Citrus aurantium* also known as the Seville orange or bitter orange. Synephrine is marketed as an ephedra substitute that increases metabolic temperature, utilizing a greater amount of fat stores as energy during a workout.   Synephrine is closely related to ephedra, increasing thermogenesis (your body's production of heat by burning fat), appetite suppression as well as increasing energy.   Although manufacturers of synephrine claim that it possesses all the beneficial characteristics of ephedra, without posing the health threats associated with ephedra, some recent data suggests that synephrine may be just as harmful as ephedra. For example, one such study found that synephrine not only causes hypertension and increases heart rate, but also interacts with other prescription medications, affecting their metabolism[41].   Metabolism of medications is the way in which your body breaks down ingested drugs so they can be eliminated from the body.   When a drug's metabolism is inhibited, toxic levels of that drug could build up in your body in a relatively short amount of time.   Synephrine may also induce vasoconstriction (narrowing of the blood vessels), leading to ischemic stroke[42]. Caffeine contaminants from guarana, maté, or other herbs in association with synephrine are thought to be responsible for the health risks associated with synephrine supplements.

Because synephrine is a dietary supplement, it is not subject to regulation by the FDA. Therefore, animal testing and clinical trials that are normally used to determine if a drug is safe are not performed. Because most dietary supplements are composed of plant materials, most supplements are contaminated with other herbs that could affect your health. It is important that you speak with your doctor before taking any dietary supplement or herbal medicine as some of them may interfere with prescription drugs and/or induce other health complications.

Although consumption of citrus juice in the morning does not increase your metabolism, citrus fruits are a good source of vitamin C as well as fiber. However, to get the beneficial effects of the fiber from citrus fruits, you must eat the fruit as a whole, not just consume the juice.

There is some evidence that certain prescription drugs interact with grapefruit juice. Such interactions usually affect the action (efficacy and safety) of those drugs, so if you take prescription drugs, consult your doctor before consuming significant amounts of grapefruit or grapefruit juice.

The best way to start burning calories at the beginning of the day is to have a well-rounded breakfast that includes some weight loss medicinal herbs and spices. The National Weight Control Registry states that eating breakfast regularly is beneficial in the long-term maintenance of weight loss[43,44]. Furthermore, eating breakfast regularly is associated with more physical activity, suggesting that consuming breakfast increases your energy.

Stress and Food Choice – Don't let it affect your weight loss

Like it or not, we all suffer the torments of stress, which usually ends with an attempt at numbing that stress with a bag of chips or a bowl of ice cream, a phenomenon called emotional eating. There are three major types of stress which vary in both duration and strength. Acute stress is the most common stress and its effects are short term. An example of acute stress may include the feeling you have following an argument with your boss, an unusually long and arduous commute to work, or bad weather. Episodic acute stress is usually found in persons suffering from nervous disorders. These people are typically known as "worry worts". Finally, there is chronic stress, typically associated with long-term troubles with little hope of resolution. Chronically stressed individuals may feel trapped, constantly surrounded by circumstances which are out of their control. Chronic stress is associated with abdominal obesity, type II diabetes, as well as cardiovascular disease and should be managed by a qualified healthcare provider. For the purposes of this article, acute stress and its relationship with food choice will be covered. If you are suffering from chronic stress or think you may be, contact your doctor immediately.

If a person is placed into a stressful situation, he or she is more likely to be subject to emotional eating. Interestingly, emotional eaters don't tend to overeat; they often eat unhealthy foods that are high in carbohydrates and/or fats. Several studies address the effects of stress on food choice, applying volunteers to various stressors then tracking which foods they selected. For example, one group of volunteers (the stressed group) was given 1 hour to prepare a 4 minute speech which they were to present after lunch while another control group (the non-stressed group) listened to a passage of 'neutral' text for 1 hour before lunch. For lunch, a variety of food choices, sweet, salty, bland, high-fat as well as low-fat food were available. Stressed volunteers, those faced with public speaking, chose more sweet and high-fat foods as compared to non-stressed control subjects[45]. Furthermore, females are more susceptible to emotional eating as compared to males[46]. These results help confirm that stress alters food choice although possibly to varying extents in males versus females.

So, why do we choose the unhealthiest foods at the least hint of a stressful situation? During stress, higher levels of stress hormones, called glucocorticoids, are secreted. Increased glucocorticoids along with consumption of comfort foods, in turn, stimulate a reorganization of energy stores from the periphery of your body to the center; hence, increasing abdominal fat deposits during stress. It is thought that increased abdominal fat suppresses the influence of stress on our emotional behavior by decreasing glucocorticoid levels, perhaps dulling our response to a particular stressor[47]. Alternatively, some comfort foods such as chocolate may stimulate the release of mood-enhancing opiates, thereby inducing a feeling of satisfaction. Finally, eating comfort foods may just be a small distraction, creating a sort of reprieve from the stressor.

Stress is a daily part of life for most people. How is a person expected to stick to any dieting regimen when faced with daily stressors? One answer is to plan ahead. Anticipating stressful situations and providing coping mechanisms is one way to ensure that you adhere to a healthy diet. For example, bringing healthy snacks to work, a typical stress-inducing environment, is one way to combat emotional eating. As with meal planning, snack planning is essential to staying within a healthy diet program.

In addition to planning ahead for potentially stress-inducing situations, tea has long been hailed for containing components that promote relaxation as well as other beneficial properties. For example, green tea (*Camella sinensis*), a popular Asian tea, just recently gaining immense popularity in the west, contains L-theanine an amino acid that when consumed has anti-anxiety properties. Also, chamomile tea, another tea that has long been used for reducing stress, decreases stress hormone production during stress[48].

Additionally, some foods provide components that combat certain side effects resulting from stress and anxiety such as lowered immune responsiveness as well as higher blood pressure. For example, vegetables such as tomato and green pepper are high in Vitamin C, an immunological booster. During stress, the high level of stress hormones represses the immune system. A recent study suggests that eating Gazpacho, a cold soup containing tomatoes, cucumbers, green peppers, onions, garlic, and olive oil, increases serum Vitamin C while decreasing stress molecules associated with vascular disease[49]. Furthermore, increasing consumption of fruits and vegetables also decreases blood pressure[50]. It should be noted that not all fruits and vegetables contribute to weight loss. Many fruits and some vegetables may indeed contribute to weight gain.

Along with planning ahead and making smart food choices, both meditation and regular exercise enable our minds and bodies to cope with stressful situations in a healthy manner. Furthermore, meditation and regular exercise both decrease blood pressure and increase confidence.

I didn't realize that stress made my tooth sweeter until I read this article. I have increased my exercise level a little and I tote my own snacks. Guess what I have in my bag today? Starts with a 'P' and ends in 'nuts'. I think I am cured.

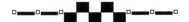

Eating for Beauty

Consuming a diet rich in beneficial nutrients such as vitamins and minerals results in many welcomed side effects such as weight loss and improved health, not to mention enhanced beauty. It is important to state here that this section is concerned with the effects of nutrients derived from certain foods (not supplements) on your overall appearance. One of the many benefits of eating more fruits and vegetables may include reduced wrinkle formation, leading to younger looking skin. The definition of a wrinkle is: a small ridge, prominence, or furrow formed by the shrinking or contraction of any smooth substance. Of course, by the shear extent of creams that exist to combat the signs of aging (i.e. wrinkles), no reader needs to be reminded of the detailed definition.

Although many of us are too familiar with the definition of a wrinkle, the reasons why we get them may not be clear. During the aging process, fat as well as collagen and elastin (matrix proteins responsible for the shape of organs) are lost in the skin. To combat wrinkle formation, many topical creams either replace the lost collagen and elastin or relax skin muscles, resulting in a smoother appearance.

Sun damage by ultraviolet radiation (UVA) is one of the leading causes of premature aging of the skin. UVA induces premature aging by generating reactive oxygen species (ROS), thereby increasing oxidative stress in the skin. ROS induced by UVA, damages lipid, DNA, and proteins located within skin cells[51]. Furthermore, UVA induces gene expression of certain enzymes, matrix metalloproteinases, which break down the support matrix, collagen and elastin, found in skin, possibly leading to wrinkle formation[51]. For this reason, many marketing ads for wrinkle creams include key words such as free radical, collagen/elastin booster, and antioxidants.

Beta-carotene is a member of the carotenoid family (the bright red, yellow, and orange pigments of fruit and vegetables) that is found in foods such as carrots and green, leafy vegetables. It is an antioxidant that is a potent ROS scavenger[52]. Because beta-carotene quenches ROS, it (ROS) can no longer damage skin lipids, proteins, and DNA. Furthermore, beta-carotene represses UVA-induced matrix metalloproteinase expression, making it one of the few oral skin protectants that fight against premature aging.

Along with directly combating premature aging by removing ROS, beta-carotene may indirectly affect wrinkle formation by increasing retinoic acid production in the skin. Beta-carotene is required for retinoic acid production which induces skin cell proliferation, perhaps leading to a thickening of the skin. In turn, a thicker skin layer may result in a smoother appearance of the surface of the skin.

Because beta-carotene eaten in the diet accumulates in the epidermis of the skin, it was tested and confirmed to aid in protecting the skin from UVA-induced premature aging[53]. Furthermore, the levels of beta-carotene obtained from a diet rich in fruits and vegetables were sufficient to produce the protection from UVA. Additionally, beta-carotene is phytoprotective (plant-derived protection) against erythema (redness of skin produced by the congestion of capillaries in the skin) induced by UVA.

To maintain the skin benefits associated with consumption of fruits and vegetables rich in beta-carotene, it is important to maintain consumption of those foods. Because UVA destroys beta-carotene in the skin, it must be replenished continuously. Keep eating your brightly-colored vegies for a younger, healthier appearance.

Have you seen the prices of wrinkle creams lately? Ouch! Please don't ask how I know these prices. With prices like that I'd rather have a wrinkle or two – they give character to the face anyway. Like most people, I am interested in slowing the aging process a little, nothing too drastic. Unlike some however, I am more interested in rejuvenating the inside – strong muscles, good joints, working kidneys, a great ticker, etc. That not withstanding, when I found out that beta carotene can fill a wrinkle or two, I paid attention to it. Nowadays I don't compromise the veggies I eat for my weekly beta carotene quota by cooking them. Try a rainbow vegetable salad on a spinach bed with an olive oil infusion of your favorite medicinal spices (next chapter). It is tasty and it fills the wrinkles. Significantly cheaper than the wrinkle creams, beta carotene will also protect you from some cancers. Of course you already knew that it is good for your vision too.

By the way, the rainbow salad is an excellent food for weight loss. Use the weight loss spices in the medicinal foods section as your dressing - i.e. grind them up and dump them in olive oil to make a tasty infusion. Cover your rainbow salad with this dressing, sprinkle a handful of nuts (almonds, peanuts, pecan nuts or walnuts) and enjoy. Feel free to visualize the beta carotene filling up your wrinkle(s) and the weight loss combo squeezing the fat out of your gut and burning it. Yes, get your mind involved so you can enjoy the maximum effects of your new found way of eating.

Red Meat and Breast Cancer- Is there a link?

Recently, it was widely reported in the news that there is a potential link between the amount of red meat that a woman consumes and her risk of developing breast cancer. While this subject may just recently be receiving some attention, researchers have been trying to formulate a potential link between nutritional intake and breast cancer risk for years. While this study is just one in many, it is the first to consider the different types of breast cancer (receptor positive versus receptor negative) and their association with red meat consumption. This article will delve into the details of this research along with discussing how red meat is thought to increase breast cancer risk.

Information from the Nurses Health Study II pertaining to red meat consumption and breast cancer was recently published [54]. The Nurses Health Study began in 1976, involving 121,700 female nurses (30-55 years of age), who filled out a questionnaire regarding their lifestyle, medical history, and overall health. Follow up questionnaires were periodically given to these same nurses along with additional nurses to better understand the connections between lifestyle and health. Subsequently, over the years, many researchers have used this data to determine whether there are connections between lifestyle and a variety of health problems.

This particular report was asking the question, "Do women, who eat more red meat, have a higher risk of developing a certain type of breast cancer than those who consume less or no red meat?" Epidemiological studies found that countries with the most animal protein consumption also had the highest rates of breast cancer, indicating that too much animal protein may be harmful [55].

Analyzing food frequency questionnaires of 90,659 women (ages 26-46) starting in 1991, the researchers reported 1021 cases of breast cancer [54]. While there was no significant correlation between red meat consumption and overall risks of breast cancer, the authors determined that women who consumed higher amounts of red meat (more than 1.5 servings of red meat/day) had a higher chance of having a certain type of breast cancer, receptor positive breast cancer [54].

What is the difference between receptor positive and receptor negative breast cancer? Firstly, the receptor that the clinicians are referring to is either estrogen receptor and/or progesterone receptor. These receptors are responsive to the female hormones estrogen and progesterone. Once these receptors are stimulated with their perspective hormone, they initiate many different functions in the cell, including cell proliferation (or multiplying) by cell division.

Because some breast cancers are more responsive to female hormones (receptor positive breast cancers), treatments to block hormone signaling called hormone therapy are common. One example of hormone therapy is tamoxifen, which binds the estrogen receptor and impedes it from sensing the circulating hormone. Thus, tumor cell proliferation can be inhibited.

Recently, researchers have noticed that the amount of receptor positive breast tumors has been on the rise, especially in pre-menopausal, middle aged women [54]. In 1992, there were 65.2 cases per 100,000 women (aged 40-49) whereas in 1998, there were 75.1 per 100,000. This observation has led many researchers to believe that environmental factors, including changes in diet, are responsible for this trend.

Although this report looks more closely at the receptor status of the breast tumors in association with red meat consumption, it should be mentioned that many previous studies did not find a link between breast cancer and red meat consumption [56,57]. One reason for this inconsistency may be preferential cooking methods.

For example, the Uruguay Study and the Iowa Women's Health Study found that fried, BBQ, or flame broiled meat consumption is linked to breast cancer risk while others indicate that stewing or boiling red meat is not [56-58]. Importantly, this association was seen in various ethnic groups with drastically different cuisines. For example, the Nurses Health Study analyzes the Western diet whereas the Shanghai Breast Cancer Study looks at a population of women who traditionally have little risk of developing breast cancer [56,58]. However, in both populations, increased charring of the meat was associated with increased breast cancer risk. Furthermore, women who consumed well done meat were 4 times more likely to develop breast cancer as compared to women that ate their meat cooked rare or medium [56].

There are many characteristics of red meat and the methods involved in its cooking that may be responsible for increasing a woman's risk of developing breast cancer. For example, charring red meat while cooking produces known mutagens, heterocyclic amines, which are carcinogenic [56,57].

Furthermore, in the U.S., cattle are still given exogenous hormones to stimulate larger growth, a practice which is banned in European countries. Because hormones may stimulate breast tumor growth, it is postulated that red meat may increase a woman's risk of breast cancer by increasing the amount of hormones to which she is exposed.

Finally, red meat and animal fats in general are typically composed of saturated and monounsaturated fatty acids while fats obtained from plants are mainly polyunsaturated and monounsaturated fats [59]. Increased fat consumption in general has been thought to be involved in breast cancer perhaps due to elevation of circulating estrogens [59].

No matter the involvement or lack thereof of red meat in breast cancer, cutting down on red meat consumption is known to prevent heart disease. That reason alone should make individuals choose to lessen their intake of red meat.

Similar clinical studies have shown a link between red meat and prostate cancer in men. As is the case with breast cancer in women, the main risk factor in prostate cancer appears to be the charring of meat. Based on this evidence, I would recommend that you take it easy on red meat, and whenever you decide to eat red meat be sure to pay attention to the cooking method. Don't overcook and avoid cooking methods that may cause charring of the meat.

Not all Fat is Created Equal

Regional fat distribution on an individual's body affects the chances of the diseases attributed to obesity. In fact, many diseases, including metabolic syndrome, heart disease and type II diabetes seem to be dependent on where your body stores excess fat rather than the amount of total body fat you may have.

You may have heard medical researchers say that an apple-shaped person is more susceptible to the disorders associated with obesity than a pear-shaped individual. What difference does it make where your body stores excess fat? Is this condition reversible? These are some of the types of questions that will be addressed in this article.

It is crucial that every overweight or obese person know whether they are apple or pear-shaped. A person that is apple-shaped stores fat in their waist area whereas a pear-shaped person stores their excess fat in the hip region.

In order to accurately determine which shape you are, first measure your waist at the narrowest point (e.g. 38 in.) and measure your hips at the widest point (e.g. 48 in.). After that, divide your waist measurement by your hip measurement (ex. 38/48). For women, a ratio greater than 0.8 means that you are apple-shaped and for men, a ratio that is 1.0 or greater indicates that you are apple-shaped. Apple-shaped individuals are more at risk of developing complications due to their weight.

To make things even more complicated, different types of fat stored in the abdominal region seem to contribute differently to obesity-associated complications. For example, epidemiological evidence indicates that it is visceral fat (fat around your internal organs) that is linked to heart disease risk factors [60]. However, there is no association between abdominal subcutaneous (skin) fat and heart disease risk.

Even in lean individuals, greater visceral fat is linked to increased risk of heart disease. For example, a study looking at 18 healthy men and 19 healthy women found that those with increased visceral fat had a higher heart disease risk profile [60]. Specifically, they had increased cholesterol levels, increased fasting glucose levels, and increased blood pressure. Obese individuals with lower amounts of visceral fat have lower risk of heart disease and type II diabetes.

In one study, individuals with Prader-Willi syndrome, (characterized by compulsive overeating, life threatening obesity, mental retardation and short stature) had overall lower visceral fat that other obese counterparts [61]. Furthermore, they had lower fasting glucose and lower triglyceride levels despite their severe obesity. Researchers believe that lower visceral fat may protect them against some of the dangerous complications associated with obesity.

Although researchers do not entirely know what determines the body fat distribution of individuals, there is some evidence that environmental factors, hormonal changes, and unfortunately genetics are all involved [61].

What makes visceral fat so dangerous? There is some evidence that visceral fat is more sensitive to signals that induce the release of free fatty acids into the blood circulation [60]. In turn, increased free fatty acid release has been linked to insulin resistance, the major hallmark in metabolic syndrome and type II diabetes. Furthermore, visceral fat typically secretes more compounds (cytokines and vasoactive peptides) that directly affect blood vessel function and therefore cardiovascular disease risk.

In severe cases, a physician may want to directly measure visceral fat by magnetic resonance imaging (MRI). Because this is a costly procedure, it is not commonly used to measure visceral fat thickness. Typically, the waist to hip ratio gives enough information for both the patient and the physician to determine the relative risk of heart disease.

So, where is the good news? Can you lose visceral fat with diet modification and exercise or is it there for good? A study of 45 abdominally obese men with high cholesterol found that diet and exercise were able to reduce their overall weight and more importantly their visceral fat [62]. Surprisingly, the men didn't have to lose much weight (approximately 11 pounds) to start changing the amount of abdominal fat that they had.

Another study of 17 overweight, sedentary men, found that exercising for 20 minutes 3 times each week for 6 weeks had a significant effect on improving insulin sensitivity [63]. That modest exercise program was also responsible for reducing visceral fat as well. All of this indicates that even modest changes in body weight by lifestyle changes will result in improving body fat composition and reduce your risk of many serious diseases.

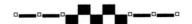

It is clear that when it comes to risk factors for health, attention should be paid to fat distribution. You must also understand that although apple-shaped individuals are more prone to certain cardiovascular diseases, pear-shaped individuals are not immune to these diseases. Being overweight in general increases your risk for these and other diseases compared to individuals who are not overweight.

The Plateau-proof diet that appears later in this book is highly effective in weight loss. As you probably already know, it is relatively more difficult to lose belly fat than it is to lose fat elsewhere in the body. The plateau-proof diet is highly effective even in making belly fat disappear. When combined with medicinal foods and weight loss herbs and spices, disease risk factors will start decreasing immediately as will body weight.

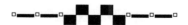

If I become a vegetarian or a vegan, will I automatically lose weight?

People switch to a vegetarian diet for many reasons including: religion, concern for animals, healthy eating and more recently weight loss. The USDA published a study of 10,014 individuals that indicated that people consuming a vegetarian diet had the lowest BMI of all the diets [64]. While many studies have shown that people who consume a vegetarian diet are less likely to be overweight or obese and that converting to a vegetarian diet may aid in weight loss, it is by no means that simple.

What do we mean by vegetarian? If you are like me, you may be wondering what composes a truly vegetarian diet since many people refer to themselves as vegetarians, but consume a wide variety of foods that others would deem "unvegetarian". A vegetarian diet is simply a dietary pattern characterized by consumption of plant foods and avoidance of some/all animal products.

For example, the most extreme vegetarians, vegans, consume a diet that includes only foods from plants such as fruits, vegetables, legumes, grains, seeds, and nuts. A vegetarian that consumes dairy products such as milk or cheese is considered a lactovegetarian whereas the ovo-lactovegetarian (or lacto-ovovegetarian) diet also includes eggs. Finally, semi-vegetarians do not eat red meat but include chicken and/or fish with plant foods, dairy products, and eggs.

Research on vegan to ovo-lactovegetarian diets indicates that each of them promote weight loss, only if done in a healthy way [64,65]. Because increased consumption of animal fat leads to increased BMI, it is no surprise that minimizing ingestion of animal fat leads to weight loss [66]. In addition to enhanced weight loss when on a vegetarian diet, vegetarians are more likely to maintain the weight loss after 5 years. Furthermore, people are more likely to stick with a vegetarian diet as opposed to other calorie restricting diets [66].

Along with enhancing weight loss, vegetarian diets may improve diabetes, particularly Type 2 diabetes in many individuals. A Seventh Day Adventist study followed 25,698 adults for 21 years and found that the incidence of diabetes (Type 1 or 2) was reduced in vegetarians compared to non-vegetarians [67]. In another study, consuming a vegetarian diet led to weight loss, reduced BMI, and decreased blood glucose levels [64,68]. In fact, vegetarians reduced their blood glucose levels by up to 28% after only 12 weeks [68].

So, how might switching to a vegetarian diet improve glycemic control in diabetics? First, vegetarians tend to consume higher amounts of fiber due to the larger portions of fruits, vegetables, legumes, etc. in their diet. Furthermore, the average person that increases their fiber intake by 14 grams each day typically reduces the total amount of energy that they consume by 10% because foods that are high in fiber tend to make you feel more full [64]. We know that even small amounts of weight reduction can significantly improve diabetes in many people.

The most exciting result was that 71% of people consuming a vegetarian diet along with engaging in moderate exercise were able to reduce their blood glucose, cholesterol, and triglyceride levels and thus reduce the amount of oral medication used to control their blood glucose [67]. These improvements were maintained up to three years after the conclusion of the study. Furthermore, insulin use was also significantly reduced.

While there are many compelling reasons to become vegetarian or at least to introduce more vegetables, fruits, nuts, and legumes into your diet, there are some precautions that you must take. Specifically, there are some nutrients such as calcium, iron, vitamin D, vitamin B12, zinc, and protein that are more abundant in animal products. You may need to take multivitamins daily to compensate for the deficiency in these vitamins and minerals. You may also consume large amounts of vegetables that are rich in these vitamins and minerals, for example;
Iron- spinach, lentils, chickpeas
Calcium- dairy products, soy, broccoli
Vitamin D- fortified milk, soy milk, or cereals
Vitamin B12- eggs, dairy, soy
Zinc- whole grain cereals, nuts, tofu, spinach
Protein- eggs, dairy products, beans, nuts, and tofu

A more comprehensive list of vegetables and their nutritional and health benefits is provided in the chapter on medicinal and health management foods.

While many studies have shown that switching to a vegetarian diet may induce or improve weight loss, you should remember that all diets require proper food choices. You can be vegetarian, choose to eat French fries smothered in cheese, and never lose a single ounce of weight. The Plateau-proof diet offers many healthy food choices, both vegetarian and non-vegetarian. These foods are carefully chosen for their weight loss potential, and for their potential to reverse the metabolic syndrome (high LDL cholesterol, low HDL cholesterol, elevated blood triglyceride levels, and elevated blood sugar levels).

A restricting vegetarian diet is likely to lead to weight loss in most people, but this weight loss may not be a robust or complete weight loss. This type of weight loss may plateau prematurely and rapid weight gain may result once diet stringency is reduced. Vitamin and mineral supplementation should be considered when you are on such a restricting diet. A vegetarian diet causes weight loss by a decrease in calories consumed. The clinique science weight loss uses many approaches to target the different weight loss parameters, rather than just calorie reduction as in a vegetarian diet. You will see these factors and how they contribute to your weight loss later. Vegetarians therefore will benefit from the clinique science weight loss for a more rapid, healthier and sustainable weight loss. When you understand the clinique science weight loss system, you will understand why you can consume more calories than another person and still lose weight faster than them.

Can a single fatty meal cause a heart attack?

Just a single meal high in saturated fats significantly affects the way your blood vessels work. A research article was published recently in the *Journal of the American College of Cardiology*, which highlights the negative effects obtained from only one meal that is high in saturated fats. After just a few hours, the ability of blood vessels to expand is reduced when eating foods high in saturated fats. Reduction in blood vessel expansion is one of the hallmarks of heart disease. Imagine what eating a diet high in saturated fats for a life time will do to your blood vessels! Now that we know that we can be severely compromising our blood vessels with just one fatty meal, immediately reducing saturated fat consumption is a must.

*I think this is an appropriate time to discuss fat – the fats that we eat. We all know what fat is, but I am still going to ask the question. **What is fat?** Fat is one of the three macronutrients that make up the bulk of the foods we eat, the other two being carbohydrate and protein. Fat is actually an important energy source for the body, with one gram of fat providing twice as much energy as one gram of carbohydrate or protein. Although fat is an essential energy source for the body, too much of the wrong type of fat in the diet may result is weight gain and/or several health problems such as heart disease and cancer. Take note that what is more important is not the amount of fat in the diet but the type of fat in the diet.*

What is the wrong type of fat and why is it bad for the body? To answer this question lets take a look at the different types of fat.

(1) **Saturated fats** are mostly derived from animal sources. Meats and whole dairy products such as milk, cream, cheese, butter and ice cream are rich in saturated fat. Saturated fat is also naturally occurring in some plant food sources such as palm kernel oil and coconut oil. This type of fat is solid at room temperature. When saturated fat is consumed, it increases blood levels of both HDL cholesterol (good cholesterol) and LDL cholesterol (bad cholesterol). These fats will cause cardiovascular disease and other diseases, therefore dietary intake must be minimized.

(2) **Trans fats** are derived from an artificial hydrogenation (of vegetable oil) process, and occur in foods such as margarine, vegetable shortening, fast food, most baked goods (especially baked goods that are sold in stores and bakeries). These fats are solid or semisolid at room temperature. Trans fats will increase the level of LDL cholesterol, lower HDL cholesterol and increase triglyceride levels when they are consumed in the diet. They will therefore cause cardiovascular and other diseases, so you should do your best to avoid trans fats.

(3) **Monounsaturated fats** occur in nuts such as almonds, cashews, peanuts and walnuts, olives, avocado, canola oil, olive oil, and peanut oil, etc. These fats are liquid at room temperature. When consumed in the diet, these fats will lower blood levels of LDL cholesterol, increase HDL cholesterol and lower triglycerides. These are therefore good fats for cardiovascular disease prevention. They will help protect you from other diseases such the type II diabetes as well.

(4) **Polyunsaturated fats** occur in fish, corn oil, soybean oil, safflower oil, and cottonseed oil. They are liquid at room temperature. Like monounsaturated fats, when consumed in the diet, polyunsaturated fats will lower blood levels of LDL cholesterol, increase HDL cholesterol and lower triglycerides. These are therefore good fats for cardiovascular disease prevention. They will help protect you from other diseases such the type II diabetes as well.

Of good and bad cholesterol

Cholesterol is an essential and important waxy compound that is mostly made by the liver, although about a quarter of total cholesterol if from our diets. Loosely speaking, there are two types of cholesterol, LDL cholesterol and HDL cholesterol. LDL (low density lipoprotein) binds cholesterol in the liver and distributes it to the rest of the body via the blood. It is referred to as bad cholesterol because it settles on and binds to the walls of the blood vessels when it is present in excess, leading to a narrowing of blood vessels and subsequently cardiovascular disease. HDL (high density lipoprotein) binds excess cholesterol in the body and returns it to the liver to be destroyed and excreted from the body. It has the opposite effect of LDL cholesterol and is therefore referred to as good cholesterol.

Food and Dyspepsia

Up to 15-20% of the Western population suffers from dyspepsia at least at some time in their life [69]. This article will discuss the types of dyspepsia, some of the causes of dyspepsia, and foods that may help alleviate the painful symptoms associated with dyspepsia. Finally, a connection between obesity and gastric ulcers will be explored.

Dyspepsia is characterized by chronic or recurrent upper abdominal pain and/or discomfort associated with gastrointestinal symptoms and a normal endoscopy (the observation of the intestines with a special camera called an endoscope). Some of the problems that can induce dyspeptic symptoms include gastroesophageal reflux, peptic ulcer disease, and gastric cancer.

Gastroesophagel reflux disease or GERD occurs when the contents of the stomach are regurgitated into the esophagus [70]. Some patients may describe GERD as heartburn. Repeated exposure of the esophagus to the digestive components of the stomach leads to esophageal inflammation and possibly cancer.

So, what causes peptic ulcers? Many peptic ulcers result from bacterial, *Helicobacter pylori (H. pylori)* infections. In fact, in the 1980s, researchers found that up to 90% of all patients with duodenal (small intestine) ulcers and 70% of patients with gastric (stomach) ulcers were infected with *H. pylori* [71]. Individuals with *H. pylori* infections tend to produce less protective mucous and secrete more gastric acid [71]. Collectively, a reduction in the protective mucous barrier and an increase in gastric acid secretion will lead to lesions in the gastrointestinal wall in many cases.

In addition to *H. pylori* infections, chronic use of nonsteroidal anti-inflammatory drugs (NSAIDs) such as aspirin is associated with the incidence of ulcers. Up to 30% of people who use NSAIDs daily will have 1 or more ulcers [71].

So, how does aspirin use trigger ulcer formation? NSAIDs affect the activity of two proteins, COX-1 and COX-2. Inhibiting COX-2 activity results in decreased pain and inflammation whereas inhibiting COX-1 activity can lead to ulcer formation. That is precisely why pharmaceutical companies have been searching for COX-2 specific inhibitors as potential pain killers that do not produce ulcers.

Is there an association between those agents that cause peptic ulcers and gastric cancer? Yes, there is an association between *H. pylori* infection and both types of gastric cancer, intestinal and diffuse. *H. pylori* infection leads to chronic inflammation, gastritis, intestinal metaplasia, dysplasia, and ultimately gastric cancer [72].

So, how does inflammation induce gastric cancer? The inflammatory process leads to oxidative stress which, in turn, damages DNA, proteins and lipids (fats). DNA damage will eventually lead to alterations in cell growth and tumor formation. In fact, curbing gastric inflammation by eradication of *H. pylori* prevents the development of pre-cancerous lesions in humans.

In addition to *H. pylori* infection, there is some evidence that diet may influence gastric cancer [72]. For example, increased consumption of fruits and vegetables is associated with decreased risk of developing gastric cancer. Furthermore, diets high in salt are associated with increased risk of gastric cancer. In fact, a high salt diet accompanied with *H. pylori* infection greatly increases the risk of developing gastric cancer.

Along with *H. pylori* infection and NSAID use, another class of peptic ulcers exists for which the cause of the ulcer is unknown. Termed idiopathic ulcers, this class of ulcers is now becoming more prevalent [73]. In an attempt to determine risk factors that lead to ulcer formation in addition to *H. pylori* infections and NSAID use, a group of Swedish researchers conducted the Kalixanda Study.

The Kalixanda Study in Sweden found that other factors including diet and fitness may influence a person's risk of developing peptic ulcers [73]. Between 1999 and 2001, this group of researchers randomly interviewed 3,000 people in two towns that had a total population of 21,610. They found that 4% of the people had peptic ulcers. Furthermore, people who smoked, used aspirin, and/or were obese had an increased risk of developing peptic ulcers.

There are several conventional therapies for dyspepsia, including: eradication of *H. pylori* infection, suppression of acid production, and/or gastrokinetic drugs that increase stomach emptying.

In addition to pharmacotherapeutic means to alleviate dyspepsia, there are some traditional medicines that may have some therapeutic benefits. For example, in Iranian folk medicine, coriander is used to relieve dyspepsia (stomach pain or discomfort including bloating, heart burn, upset stomach, and belching).

If you have dyspepsia you now know that you have to eat a good load of vegetables to avoid further complications such as gastric cancer. The herbs and vegetables that may help protect you from gastric cancer are listed in the medicinal and health management foods chapter. Healthcare professionals often recommend eating fruits and vegetables without specifying which. This is a dangerous and irresponsible practice because not all fruits and vegetables are good for you, especially if you are trying to lose weight. The plateau-proof diet section arranges fruits and vegetables (along with other foods) in tables so that you know which to eat for weight loss and which to avoid. The plateau-proof diet goes further to assign numbers to all foods, with smaller numbers being good for weight loss and larger numbers being bad. Back to the topic at hand, adding coriander to your food may help relieve dyspepsia. Also see the medicinal foods section.

Are you what you drink? The effects of soft drink consumption on weight

What people eat and how that affects their weight tends to be the major focus of the popular weight loss diets and weight loss research. However, beverages make up approximately 21% of a person's total energy intake. Does drinking an occasional sweetened beverage really contribute to weight gain? This article will discuss the research surrounding sweetened beverage consumption, particularly with respect to soft drinks and their effects on BMI, to help you make informed choices concerning the contents of the next glass that you bring to your mouth.

It is no surprise to learn that people in general are consuming more soft drinks than they were 20 years ago. On average, people are consuming 150-300 kcalories more than they were just 10 years ago, half of which comes from soft drinks [74]. In 2001 for example, the average person consumed 3 times more soft drinks than they did in 1977. Not only has the amount of soft drinks that we consume increased, but the portion size that we drink is also larger, increasing from 13.6 oz to 21 oz. The fact that increased consumption of soft drinks coincided with the current obesity epidemic has led some researchers to ask whether increased soft drink consumption could be responsible at least in part for the current rise in obesity.

Multiple studies have addressed the importance of making proper beverage choices and the effects to a person's weight gain when they continually drink sweetened beverages such as soft drinks. The findings show that these sweetened drinks are causing weight gain. Not only is this affecting your weight but it is contributing to your children's weight gain as well.

On average, children in the U.S. drink the equivalent of 2 cans of soda per day, accounting for approximately 5.5% of the total energy that they consume each day. Multiple studies indicate that kids who drink soft drinks more than once per day are more likely to have higher BMIs than kids who drink soda less than once a week. Additionally, a significant drop in obesity was seen in kids that reduced their soft drink intake [75].

How might frequent soft drink consumption lead to higher BMI? First, soft drinks are loaded with calories and their glycemic index is also quite high. Furthermore, soft drinks are not satiating (the feeling of fullness), resulting in the feeling of hunger and consequently more food intake. Finally, consumption of sweetened beverages replaces consumption of more healthy beverages, such as water and unsweetened tea.

In addition to likely weight gain, kids that frequently drink soft drinks are less likely to drink milk and thereby have low calcium levels. In fact, milk consumption in kids has collectively decreased by 25% in the last 10 years [76]. Concern for developing osteoporosis later in life is just another consequence of frequent soft drink consumption. In addition, milk provides other nutrients such as protein, zinc, vitamin A and vitamin C that are reduced in kids that replace milk with soft drinks.

As a result of these studies, restrictions in soft drink advertising to children and removal of vending machines that sell soft drinks in schools have occurred. Despite these restrictions, the School Health Policies and Programs Study found that of the school districts interviewed, 49.9% of them had soft drink contracts and 2/3 of the schools were given incentives to increase their sales

[77].   Furthermore, 1/3 of the schools permitted soft drink advertisements.

Children are not the only group whose weight is affected by soft drink consumption. An association between increased soft drink consumption with increased BMI is also seen in adults. In just 10 weeks of drinking soft drinks, a group of overweight adults gained an average of 3.5 pounds (1.6 kg) while a control group, which drank artificially sweetened beverages actually lost 2.2 pounds (1 kg) [78]. In addition, another study found that women who increased their soft drink consumption from 1 or less soft drink per week to 1 or more soft drinks per day gained an average of over 10 pounds (~5 kg) [79]. The same study determined that women who drank one or more soft drinks per day increased their chances of developing Type II diabetes by 80% whereas women who drank diet sodas had no increased risk [79].

Are diet soft drinks the answer? Much of the research surrounding soft drink consumption has compared it to consumption of diet sodas. Although the weight gain associated with soft drinks is not seen with diet sodas, there is still a concern in replacing nutritious beverages with beverages that offer no nutritious value such as diet soft drinks.

It is also important to consider that soft drinks are not the only reason for today's obesity epidemic. In addition to eating more and more energy rich foods, we are moving considerably less. There are also other important factors responsible for obesity and weight gain that are discussed elsewhere in this book. So, although cutting down on your intake of sweetened beverages such as soft drinks will get you started, it is by no means the only answer to your weight problems.

One of the unique features of the Plateau-proof Diet compared to other popular diets is that it considers not only the foods that you eat, but also the beverages that you drink. Consequently, you can find most of your favorite beverages within the green, yellow, and red tables. Soft drinks consumption is not recommended while following the Plateau-proof diet since soft drinks are located in the red tables of both CP and FP rotations.

Beverage Guidance Council's suggested beverage consumption pattern:
- Water 50 oz
- Tea/Coffee 28 oz
- Low fat milk 16 oz
- No calorie sweetened beverage 0-32 oz
- Caloric beverages with nutrients (alcohol/fruit juice) 0-8 oz
- Caloric beverages without nutrients (soda) 0-8 oz

American Beverage Association's guidelines for beverage availability in schools:
- **Elementary schools**- water and 100% juice
- **Middle schools**- water, 100% juice, sports drinks, no-calorie soft drinks, and low calorie juice drinks
- **High schools**- water, 100% juice, sports drinks, no-calorie soft drinks, and low calorie juice drinks. They also propose that no more than 50% of the vending selections be soft drinks.

The Plateau-proof Diet scrutinizes each type of juice individually. Some juices may be as harmful as sodas because of their high content of naturally occurring sugars.

For some people this is where the weight loss battle is won or lost – drinks. If I was raised by wolves and therefore a stranger to the human condition, my advice would simply be to eliminate all drinks that have a sweet taste (e.g. sodas), all drinks that contain sodium (e.g. sports drinks) and all drinks that contain saturated fats (milk and other dairy drinks). I would be right on the money with that advice because making those cuts will facilitate your weight loss, and improve your cardiovascular health. That will leave you with teas, water, and fat-free milk. Being a member of this civilization, I realize that most people will have a tough time giving up sweetened drinks. Orange soda was my weakness at some point in history that seems so distant at this moment. I had to wean myself off the enticing taste and flavor of orange soda by progressively diluting it with water over a period of a couple of weeks – up to the point where there was barely enough soda in the water to slightly color it. I was then ready to enjoy water for the beautiful drink that it is. I recommend this approach if you are in love with soda as I was and are unable to give it up cold turkey.

*If you would like to lose a lot of weight fast, then you should brew my potent herbal weight loss tea (See the recipe in Chapter 2), and either enjoy it hot or chill it and enjoy it as an iced tea. This is an inexpensive recipe that was very effective for weight loss in a limited clinical trial. It is simply a combination of two naturally occurring foods, each of which has very little effect on weight loss but become potent when combined. You probably already have the two foods in your garden, and if not they are inexpensive in the market. I hope they remain inexpensive now that the secret is out. In addition to my herbal tea, regular teas such as green tea and some herbal teas may improve or maintain certain health parameters, and also help protect you from disease. If you must sweeten your tea, please use a sugar-free sweetener.

Sports drinks and many other soft drinks contain sodium. Sodium is a component of the salt that we season our food with. Reducing the amount of sodium (including salt) in our diet may contribute to weight loss by impairing the absorption of sugar from the intestine. Also, it may lead to a lowering of blood pressure and improved cardiovascular health. Milk other than fat-free milk fails to make the cut of allowed beverages for the plateau-proof diet. As you read earlier, milk and other dairy products are rich in saturated fats, and now we know that a single serving of saturated fats may set your health backwards. In fact, saturated fats may slow down the metabolism of carbohydrates and fats, leading to weight gain and perhaps type II diabetes and cardiovascular disease.

*Please note that I am not claiming that my herbal tea is a magic recipe for weight loss. Although it helps in weight loss you will have to follow all of the advice and directives provided in this book to experience a complete, healthy, and sustainable weight loss.

Does alcohol have a role in obesity and weight loss?

While we are talking about beverages and weight loss, this is an appropriate time to discuss the role of alcohol in weight loss and/or weight gain. Several clinical studies have shown that moderate consumption of alcoholic beverages may be beneficial for cardiovascular health. Does moderate consumption of alcohol also help with weight loss? Although most diet programs discourage the consumption of alcoholic beverages, moderate consumption of alcohol may actually be beneficial for weight loss. At least one clinical study has shown that moderate consumption of wine does not affect the outcome of weight loss during dieting[2]. Another study involving 334 identical twins showed that the moderate alcohol consuming siblings were leaner than the siblings who abstained from alcohol[3]. Other studies have suggested that consumption of alcohol may contribute to weight loss or may prevent weight gain[4,5].

Alcohol is a slippery slope however, as excessive consumption of alcohol may cause obesity[6] and other health problems. In some people, excessive consumption of alcohol may lead to weight loss due to malnutrition[7]. I do not recommend alcohol as a facilitator of weight loss. If you are already a moderate consumer of alcohol, you may not need to change your drinking habits to enjoy the full benefits of the clinique science system. If you do not drink alcohol, there is no need to start drinking now. There are many medicinal foods that may give you a better cardiovascular profile as well as facilitate your weight loss.

Does consumption of dairy increase weight loss?

Unfortunately, the answer to this 'dieting tip' is not so clear. The simplest answer is that some studies find that increasing your intake of calcium through consumption of dairy products increases an individual's weight loss while other studies find that there is no difference. Finally, to really confuse an individual, still other studies find that increased milk consumption in children may actually predict the likelihood that your child will be overweight. So, which studies are true?

Numerous observational studies (e.g. NHANES and the Quebec Family Study) have highlighted an inverse relationship between dietary calcium and/or dairy intake and body fat or obesity. That is, a person who consumes less dairy is more likely to be overweight or obese [80].

Smaller and more controlled studies (less variables) using obese adults indicate that individuals on a calorie restricted diet while consuming more dairy lose more weight than individuals on a calorie restricted diet that consumed either low dairy or calcium supplements [81]. In a study 32 obese adults were split into three groups each consuming a calorie restricted diet with one modification 1) high calcium obtained from 3-4 servings of dairy/day, 2) high calcium, low dairy obtained from calcium supplements, and 3) low calcium, low dairy. A serving size for dairy products includes 8 oz. milk, 1 cup of yogurt, 1.5 oz. hard cheese or 2 oz. processed cheese.

After 24 weeks, the heights and weights of the individual groups were measured and the researchers determined that both groups 1 and 2 lost more weight than the low calcium and low dairy group.   Furthermore, the group that obtained their calcium through ingestion of dairy lost even more weight than those who used calcium supplements. This indicates that dairy foods may contain other unknown factors that aid in weight loss in addition to calcium.   Additionally, the high dairy group lost more abdominal fat, which is linked to many complications including heart disease.   Also, a subsequent study of 34 obese adults found that consumption of yogurt (3 servings of 6 oz. each) as the main source of dietary calcium also resulted in enhanced weight loss [80].

So how does calcium increase a person's chances of losing weight?   Some research has determined that calcium may actually help your fat cells breakdown fat.   Furthermore, dairy products also contain other minerals such as magnesium and phosphorus that may enhance the breakdown of fat by calcium. Also, dairy products are high in protein which could increase metabolism while preserving muscle mass [82].

Although these studies indicate that increased dairy consumption may lead to enhanced weight loss in obese individuals, the number of study participants was small and the study was relatively short.   Furthermore, both studies used a specific population of obese individuals, which may not reflect the effects of calcium/dairy consumption on the population as a whole. Finally, the participants in this study were on a calorie restricted diet in conjunction with consuming dairy or not. This does not tell us anything about the effects of dairy consumption in people of different ages who are consuming normal diets.

In fact, a report by Berkey and colleagues indicates that children who consume more than 3 servings of milk/day are more likely to be overweight [83]. In the Growing Up Today study, 12,829 children between the ages of 9-14 answered questionnaires concerning the types of food they ate. Children who consumed over 3 servings of milk/day were more likely to have a higher BMI. Interestingly, the correlation between milk consumption and BMI was similar whether the kids drank low fat milk or whole milk.

So, what's the take home message? Until we know more details concerning dairy and weight loss or weight gain in a variety of individuals of various ages, it is recommended that you don't start guzzling milk in the hopes of losing some extra pounds. The U.S. Department of Agriculture's Food Guide Pyramid recommends 2-3 servings of dairy products per day. My advice is not to exceed this recommended amount.

Dairy foods including beverages are considered in the Plateau-proof Diet. Nonfat milk and yogurt are found in the Green Tables in both the CP and the FP rotations (allowed). However, cheese, 1%, 2%, and whole milk are found in the Red Tables in both CP and FP rotations (not allowed).

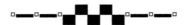

Garlic – A food for your heart and for your mind

Garlic may perhaps be one of the oldest natural medicinal foods known to man. In fact, evidence for the utilization of garlic as a natural remedy for a variety of illnesses has been found buried in tombs and temples as well as in medical texts from a variety of ancient cultures in India, Egypt, Rome, China and Japan [84,85]. Actually, garlic may have been the first known performance-enhancing agent used in the first Olympic Games. Until today, garlic is still commonly used as a medicinal food being the most popular herbal supplement in the single herb category. This article will discuss the possible uses of garlic bulbs (not supplements) as a medicinal food for heart disease as well as dementia.

Garlic is derived from the bulbs of the herb, *Allium sativum.* It is commonly used to flavor many dishes from around the world. Furthermore, in traditional medicines, garlic is used for the treatment of gastrointestinal disorders, heart problems, worms, wound healing, etc [86].

Epidemiological studies (studies involving the distribution of health-related issues within certain populations) indicate that there is inverse correlation between garlic consumption and heart disease as well as some cancers (gastric and colorectal cancer), indicating that those who include more garlic in their diet are less likely to develop these illnesses [86,87]. Furthermore, laboratory studies indicate that garlic consumption reduces the risk of developing heart disease.

Risk factors for heart disease include high cholesterol, hypertension (high blood pressure), inflammation, obesity and smoking.   Studies indicate that garlic consumption decreases cholesterol levels perhaps by reducing cholesterol production [86]. Along with reducing cholesterol levels, garlic may reduce blood pressure as well as inhibit platelet aggregation, decreasing clot formation [86].   Decreased serum cholesterol, lower blood pressure, and reduction of platelet aggregation collectively can reduce your risk of heart disease.

Some of the risk factors for heart disease such as high cholesterol, blood pressure and inflammation also increase a person's risk for developing dementias such as Alzheimer's disease [88].   High serum cholesterol levels can lead to plaque formation in blood vessels, leading to either a heart attack or stroke. When a person has a stroke, parts of the brain may not be adequately supplied with oxygen due to disruption of proper blood flow, leading to neuronal death that could produce dementias. Furthermore, high cholesterol and blood pressure is also associated with increased levels of Beta-amyloid, a hallmark of Alzheimer's disease.

So, how does garlic reduce your risk for dementia?   Because garlic reduces cholesterol levels as well as blood pressure in individuals, it may prevent neuronal damage brought on by strokes [88].   Also, garlic is high in antioxidants which also fight both heart disease and neuronal death.   In fact, there is some evidence that garlic consumption may actually improve learning and memory retention in some individuals.

Although many studies illustrate the health benefits associated with garlic consumption, some do not. These discrepancies may be explained by the fact that some studies use garlic supplements instead of whole, raw or cooked garlic. Analysis of a host of garlic supplements highlights the fact that there are many differences between them. Not only are there differences in the efficacy (the ability of a drug to control or cure an illness) between garlic supplements but there are also major differences in toxicity.

So, why are there huge differences in garlic supplements? In fact, these discrepancies are not just found in garlic supplements but indicative of supplements in general. Garlic is a food which like all foods consists of a unique chemical composition. Different processing techniques yield different garlic products including garlic essential oil, garlic powder, and aged garlic extract (AGE).

Some products such as garlic powder do not lower blood cholesterol levels [89]. Furthermore, there is some evidence that ingestion of high levels of garlic powder may interfere with drug metabolism (the way in which your body breaks down ingested drugs before they can be eliminated from the body) [89].

AGE is the most commonly used and studied garlic supplement. AGE is produced by extracting the garlic for more than 10 months, resulting in a less harsh and irritating taste and odor. Because excessive garlic consumption may be irritating to some people causing stomach problems such as a burning sensation and diarrhea, some individuals prefer AGE to raw garlic. However, as with all processing techniques, some components, which may be responsible for some of the health benefits of that food, are lost during the preparation.

So, to ensure you receive all the health benefits of garlic consumption without the worries of contaminants and safety issues, it is recommended that individuals consume whole or crushed (minced) garlic in foods instead of taking garlic supplements.

> *Only about a quarter of our blood cholesterol comes from the foods we eat. Most of the cholesterol in our blood comes from the liver where it is made. Reducing the amount of saturated fats in the diet may therefore not be enough to reduce blood cholesterol to safe levels. Since garlic and other cholesterol-reducing foods (see the medicinal foods section) may reduce cholesterol by decreasing its production, they should be vital components of your diet if your blood cholesterol levels are not in check. The plateau-proof diet has two sections – a regular plateau-proof diet and a plateau-proof diet cardio. The plateau-proof diet cardio is lower in saturated fats and higher in fiber than the regular plateau-proof diet. If your cholesterol level is not in check you should follow the plateau-proof diet cardio.*

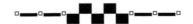

Does consumption of spicy, chili pepper help in weight loss?

Let's put it this way, if you think that you will lose weight just by chomping on some jalapeño or other tasty chili peppers alone, you are mistaken. However, there are some reports that seem to indicate that consumption of chili pepper may induce thermogenesis, increase metabolism and increase satiety (the feeling of fullness). Each of these characteristics aid in weight loss; however, as we consider the details of those reports, it is difficult to conclude if the general population will also receive the same benefits.

Chili pepper is the fruit of the *Capsicum* species of perennial plants. Red, chili pepper is used in a variety of foods including meats, seafood, and pickles in Indian, Mexican, and Caribbean cuisines. One of the active components of chili peppers, collectively called capsaicinoids, has been well studied for its health benefits. Capsaicin is the component of chili peppers that offer the special pungency well known to chili peppers while capsiate is the non-pungent capsaicinoid derived from sweet pepper.

Along with adding some spice to your meal, increased consumption of capsaicin via chili peppers may enhance satiety, resulting in suppressed food intake. In addition, it may enhance energy metabolism and modify your macronutrient intake, resulting in reduced body fat mass and decreased fat consumption, respectively [90,91]. However, upon closer inspection of those reports supporting increased chili pepper consumption for weight loss, it is clear that the experiments were short-term and contained very few participants.

For example, in one study, a total of 13 Japanese men either ate a spicy or bland breakfast [92]. Men that consumed the spicy breakfast reported less hunger after breakfast and ate less protein and fat during lunch. However, this was a one day study of a particularly small, homogeneous population. Another small study of 8 male, long distance runners indicated that consumption of spicy food may increase resting metabolic rates in humans [93]. However, once the men started exercising, there was no difference in the metabolic rates between those who had a spicy breakfast versus those who ate the bland breakfast.

Another report looked at whether capsaicin consumption aids in the maintenance of body weight after weight loss. This report, while considerably larger than the other two (91 moderately obese individuals), found that capsaicin did not improve an individual's weight loss, nor did it protect an individual from the dreaded weight gain after discontinuing a diet [5]. This either indicates that capsaicin does not enhance weight loss in general or capsaicin doesn't aid in weight loss in larger individuals.

Although chili pepper consumption is not likely to boost your weight loss, it has been used in traditional medicines and does seem to have additional health benefits in some individuals. For example, red chili pepper is used as a treatment for diabetes in Jamaican folk medicine. Subsequent analysis of the validity of that traditional medicine revealed that the active component of red pepper, capsaicin, stimulates insulin release as well as stabilizing blood glucose levels [94,95]. Additionally, in Mayan traditional medicine, red chili pepper was used as a treatment for a variety of ailments that were most likely caused by bacterial infections such as bowel disorders, ear aches, infected wounds and fresh burns. Subsequent analysis of a variety of chili peppers found that most possess antimicrobial activity [96]. This anti-microbial activity is probably why chili peppers are one of the world's most common preservative.

Although hot peppers may contribute only modestly to weight loss, eating them with other medicinal foods on a regular basis may lead to a more significant weight loss.

An important take home message here is that there is not a single miracle potion for weight loss. Rather, when medicinal herbs and spices are combined creatively and used as food seasonings or teas, things such as hot peppers which may have very little effect on weight loss may become decent weight loss facilitators. A good example again is my herbal weight loss formula, where two natural foods with little individual effect on weight loss become potent weight loss facilitators when combined.

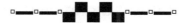

Chocolate – No Longer Just a Comfort Food

No doubt, many chocolate lovers may have been pleased to hear the news alluding to certain health benefits derived from chocolate consumption. No longer just a mid-afternoon pick-me-up, but possibly a weight loss inducer, cancer preventor, and heart healthy snack, chocolate may just be that tasty miracle we have been longing. This article will consider research studies pertaining to chocolate consumption and heart disease and help determine if all the hype is warranted or just wishful thinking.

Let us begin with a brief history of chocolate and its uses in traditional medicines from early meso-America to 17th and 18th century Europe. Chocolate or cocoa has been used for medicinal purposes for a long while, providing a tasty remedy for a variety of ailments including low sexual desire and heart pain [97]. In fact, until just recently chocolate was viewed as much more than a comfort food.

Along with historical uses of cocoa in early meso-America, recent studies of an indigenous population of Native Americans, the Kuna Indians of Panama, has shed light on some of the benefits of cocoa consumption [98]. Specifically, the Kuna people in general have almost no incidence of hypertension (high blood pressure). However, when the Kuna move to urban Panama City, the incidence of hypertension is elevated, indicating that the protective mechanism is not genetic but environmental (lifestyle habits).

So, what are the differences in lifestyle between rural and urban Kuna? Among the probable factors, rural Kuna consume a diet rich in fruits and vegetables along with fish, and city dwelling

Kuna don't eat as much fish. Furthermore, rural Kuna ingest a traditional drink that contains large amounts of cocoa that they themselves prepare. While urban Kuna continue to consume the traditional beverage, the cocoa that is used is obtained from local stores. Detailed analysis of the two cocoas revealed huge disparities in flavonoid (anti-oxidant) content between the cocoas.

So, what are flavonoids? Flavonoids are a class of anti-oxidant components found in many foods such as cocoa bean, fruits, vegetables, tea, and red wine. Of the bunch, cocoa has the highest quantity of the flavonoids (epicatechin, catechin, and procyanidins). It is these flavonoids that give chocolate its characteristic bitter flavor. Furthermore, dark chocolate has almost 2.5 times more flavonoids than milk chocolate, and white chocolate has virtually no flavonoids.

Consumption of foods high in flavonoids has long been correlated with decreased risk of developing heart disease and dying from it. Nevertheless, we saw with the Kuna story that not all chocolate products contain flavonoids. Where do they go?

While there may be differences in flavonoid concentrations due to genetic contributions from the plants themselves as well as general farming practices, the major cause for diverse flavonoid concentrations between chocolate-containing products comes from the processing and manufacturing of the cocoa bean, which can potentially result in a 90% loss of flavonoids. Specifically, fermentation and roasting of the cocoa bean cause major losses in flavonoid concentrations. Furthermore, a process called alkalization, a treatment used to remove the bitterness of the cocoa bean, also causes loss of flavonoids. Finally, there is evidence that addition of dairy products such as milk to produce milk chocolate may decrease the antioxidant properties of the cocoa [99].

Just how do flavonoids help protect you against heart disease? During the progression of heart disease, a lot of oxidative damage occurs. That damage may be responsible for platelet aggregation (clot formation), and oxidized lipids such as LDL cholesterol (bad cholesterol) are involved in atherosclerosis possibly by sticking to the wall of blood vessels and restricting blood flow. Additionally, chocolate consumption may lower your blood pressure and increase production of vasodilators [100]

At this point, you may be confused as to how a food high in fat and sugar might actually lower your risk of heart disease when many similar energy-rich foods can lead to obesity and heart disease. It is true that approximately half the weight of a cocoa bean is from cocoa butter, the fat found in chocolate that is responsible for its ability to smoothly melt [97]. Even more puzzling, cocoa butter is composed of mixture of fats, half of which are saturated (bad fats) [100]. Stearic acid, the main saturated fat in cocoa butter, is an unusual saturated fat in that it doesn't increase blood lipid levels as other saturated fats do, and it may actually protect against heart disease [100].

In case you are wondering why stearic acid, being a saturated fat, does not contribute to heart disease, you are not alone. Research along with some scientific guesstimation indicate that perhaps the body just doesn't absorb stearic acid as well as some of the other saturated fats, so it doesn't get anywhere to really do any harm. The other possibility is that the body converts stearic acid to an unsaturated fat, oleic acid. Although neither of these possibilities has been entirely proven, consumption of stearic acid-containing foods seems to have very little effect on blood lipid levels nonetheless.

Along with being one of the richest sources of antioxidants, chocolate is also a good source of minerals. For example, dark chocolate can provide up to 15% of your daily recommended amount of magnesium and 34% of your daily recommended amount of copper.

So, like most people, you may be quite anxious to find out how much chocolate you have to "force" down to get the heart healthy benefits that chocolate seems to provide. This answer is never straightforward. While there is a growing amount of evidence that points to chocolate consumption lowering your risk for heart disease, a long term study of the benefits of chocolate consumption has not been completed. Furthermore, the flavonoid concentration varies greatly from chocolate to chocolate, and because flavonoid concentrations are not labeled on chocolate products, the consumer has no way of knowing which brand offers the most antioxidant potential. Until further studies are performed, moderate consumption of dark chocolate does not seem to pose any serious threats, and could rather be helpful in warding off heart disease.

Another possible mechanism of action of dark cocoa is the disruption of fat metabolism[1]. There are two components of fat metabolism – the first breaks down fat and burns it to provide energy for the body while the other builds up fat and stores it in fat cells. Dark cocoa blocks the part of metabolism that builds and stores fat, thereby helping in weight loss. Essentially all of the three macronutrients that make up the bulk of our food (carbohydrate, fat, and protein) can be stored as fat in fat cells. Both carbohydrate and protein can be converted to fat in the body. The body does not store carbohydrates and proteins for the long term, so excess carbohydrates and proteins that we eat get converted into fat and stored. With protein, the liver can also destroy the excess and excrete it from the body. This is one of several reasons why protein is good for weight loss, compared to carbohydrate. This doesn't mean that you should eliminate all carbohydrate from your diet. Rather, as you will see in the plateau-proof diet section of this book, there are actually some carbohydrates that will facilitate your weight loss. Metabolism charts are included in the next few pages. They are only provided as a reference, in case you are interested in the details of metabolism. You don't need to understand these charts to properly follow the clnique science weight loss system.

Dark cocoa also increases thermogenesis. That is, body temperature (hence energy consumption) is increased when dark cocoa is eaten. This mechanism of action is complementary to the earlier discussed mechanism, and will also contribute to weight loss.

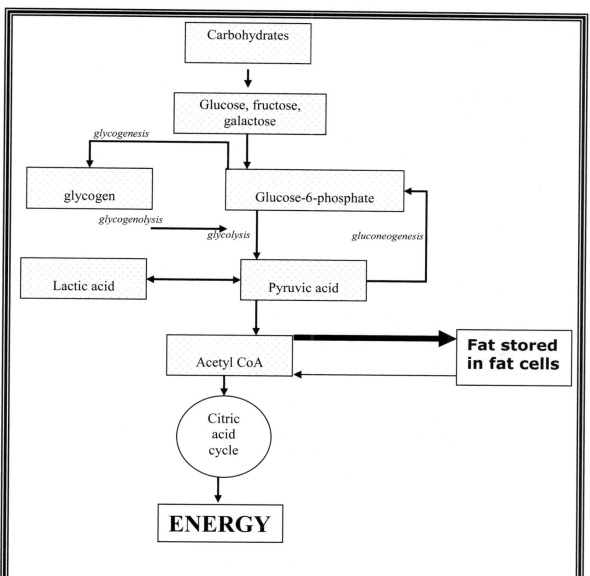

<u>Figure 1. Summary of carbohydrate metabolism.</u> *The carbohydrates that we eat are digested into three simple sugars glucose, fructose and galactose which are absorbed into the bloodstream from the intestines. All three simple sugars are then converted to a form of glucose called glucose-6-phosphate. Glucose-6-phosphate when in excess can be converted into glycogen for short term storage. If there is the need for energy glucose-6-phosphate is converted to a series of intermediaries and finally to Acetyl CoA which is burnt to produce energy. If there is more glucose-6-phosphate than is required to meet the energy demands of the body Acetyl CoA is not burnt to produce energy, rather it is converted into fat and stored in fat cells.*

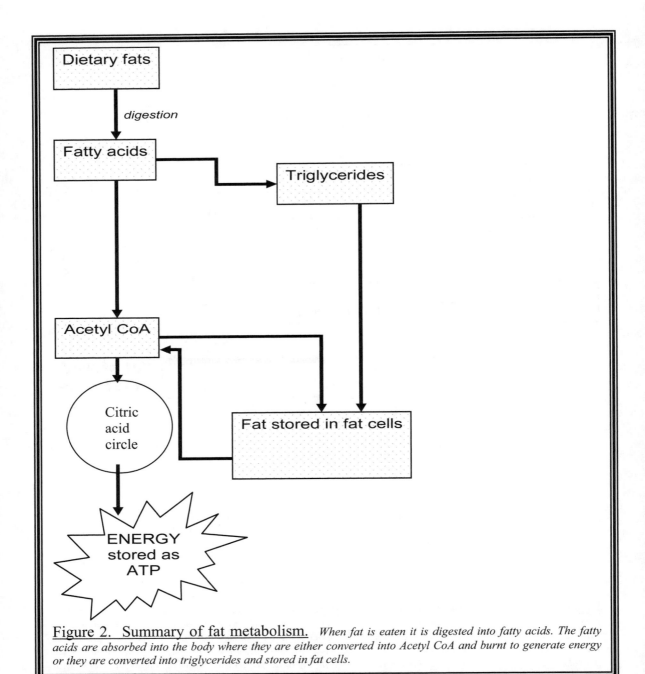

Figure 2. Summary of fat metabolism. *When fat is eaten it is digested into fatty acids. The fatty acids are absorbed into the body where they are either converted into Acetyl CoA and burnt to generate energy or they are converted into triglycerides and stored in fat cells.*

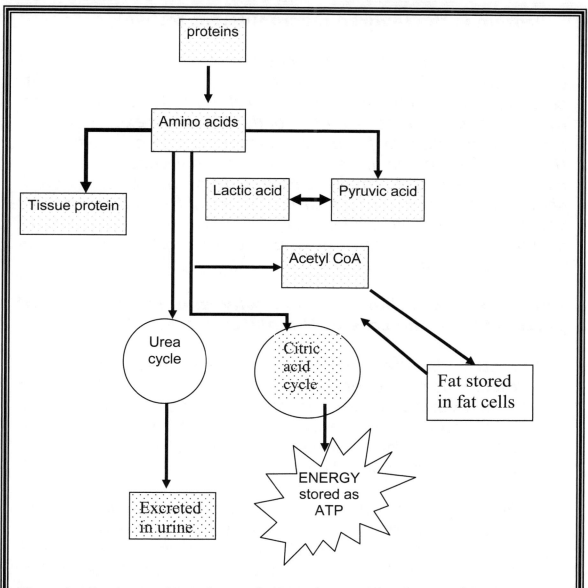

Figure 3. Summary of protein metabolism. *The proteins we eat are digested into amino acids which are absorbed into the body. The amino acids are used to build and maintain our body. They may also be used for energy or converted into fats – although not as readily as carbohydrates and fats. Excess protein is normally broken down in the liver and excreted from the body.*

Protein is the favored macronutrient for weight loss

The summary of metabolism shows that of the foods we eat, excess carbohydrates and fats are readily stored as fat in fat cells. Excess protein is however preferentially destroyed by the liver and excreted from the body. Although excess protein can be converted to fat under certain conditions, this is not the preferred metabolic route under normal conditions. Since excess protein is normally excreted from the body, protein should form the core of a sustainable weight loss diet. For this reason and other reasons stated below, the right types of proteins form the core of the plateau-proof diet that is discussed later in this book.

Here are the other reasons why the right types of proteins form the core of the plateau-proof diet:

1) Protein is the only macronutrient that has normal metabolism in obesity. The metabolism of both fat and carbohydrate is compromised and deficient. That is, the body tends to be inefficient at burning carbohydrate and fat and therefore increasing amounts of fat are stored in fat cells during obesity.

2) Protein triggers thermogenesis shortly after it is eaten. The body burns energy as heat during the process of thermogenesis. In the absence of thermogenesis, this energy would be stored as fat in the body. Since neither carbohydrates nor fats induce thermogenesis, it is not such a bright idea swallowing them down without the right types of proteins.

3) Protein may trigger the secretion of growth hormone during weight loss. Growth hormone secretion is essential to maintain a lean body in adults. When we gain weight the secretion of growth hormone is compromised, and the blood level of growth hormone drops. Weight loss by itself may not trigger the release of growth hormone; however, weight loss on a high-protein diet may trigger release of growth hormone. It is easier to lose weight and maintain a lean look when growth hormone is present in the blood.

4) Proteins may increase the rate of burning of stored fat. Studies have shown that high protein in the diet has a direct effect on increasing the rate of breakdown of fat that is stored in fat cells.

5) A high-protein weight loss diet is particularly effective in decreasing gut (visceral) fat. This is very important for cardiovascular health because gut fat is a significant risk factor for cardiovascular disease.

6) Diets rich in protein affect satiety (feeling of fullness) faster, hence minimizing the risk of overeating.

7) Protein rich diets are safe for long-term use. Studies have shown that substituting certain carbohydrates and fats for proteins leads to an improved health profile.

8) Diets rich in the right types of proteins may lower blood glucose, triglyceride, and LDL cholesterol levels and increase HDL cholesterol levels.

The Winter Blues and Weight Gain

Seasonal affective disorder (SAD), otherwise known as winter depression or the winter blues, affects 4-10% of the population, occurring most commonly in women [101]. SAD is characterized by severe mood changes as well as changes in energy and appetite, resulting in depression, fatigue, low libido, increased carbohydrate consumption, and thus weight gain.

So, what is SAD? To be diagnosed with SAD, the above mentioned symptoms will only occur in the fall and winter seasons. In the spring and summer months, those symptoms recede and in some individuals, may be replaced by manic (excitement of psychotic proportions manifested by mental and physical hyperactivity, disorganized behavior, and elevation of mood) characteristics during the summer months.

SAD can also vary in severity from individual to individual. In fact, there are two sub-categories of SAD, which are characterized by milder symptoms [101]. First, there is a sub-syndral form of SAD in which the symptoms of SAD are milder although still clinically relevant. In addition to sub-syndral SAD, there is seasonality, which is the mildest form of SAD. Seasonality is characterized by reduced performance of an individual in the winter months as compared to the summer.

What causes SAD? Some researchers and clinicians believe that shorter days and drops in the temperature serve as an evolutionary reminder that it is time to gather food for the winter, a time of the year in which individuals are less active. Although this hypothesis is difficult to test, we do know that changes in daylight affect our general mood and behavior [102]. Other, more substantive theories surrounding SAD include low serotonin and high melatonin levels.

Serotonin and melatonin are both chemical messengers (neurotransmitters) that are made in the brain. Serotonin production in the brain affects emotions and behavior. Serotonin is converted to melatonin in the brain in response to darkness. Melatonin is thought to be a key regulator of circadian rhythms. Individuals with SAD have higher levels of melatonin, possibly due to shorter daylight hours in the winter, and subsequently have reduced serotonin levels [101]. Decreased serotonin levels are known to induce hyperphagia (overeating) and cravings for carbohydrates as well as depression.

So, how do you treat SAD? The most common treatment for SAD is light therapy [101]. Although the way in which light therapy works is not fully known, research has shown that light therapy (usually 2 hours/day) suppressed the production of melatonin. Furthermore, light therapy is beneficial in up to 70% of individuals suffering SAD. Additionally, there are little to no side effects associated with light therapy. The only negative aspect of light therapy involves the amount of time each day that is required for treatment. To address this issue, a research group in Switzerland asked if patients exposed to natural light (during a morning walk) can obtain the same benefits of artificial light therapy. Indeed, the people exposed to natural light reported reduced symptoms of SAD, including less time sleeping, increased activity, and less carbohydrate consumption.

In addition to light therapy, other treatments for SAD have been examined, including ingestion of L-tryptophan and St. John's wort (*Hypericum perforatum*). In one study, individuals suffering from SAD were given the serotonin precursor, L-tryptophan (2 grams), two to three times per day or subjected to light therapy. SAD symptoms were reduced with both treatments similarly (3).

Because consumption of St. John's wort may relieve depression in some individuals, researchers asked, 'Could it also be used to treat SAD?' Two studies comparing St. John's wort (900 mg/day) with light therapy determined that both equally aided in reducing the symptoms associated with SAD, including reduced depression, fatigue, and anxiety [103]. Although St. John's wort has been used in many traditional medicines for excitability, anxiety, and depression, a cautionary note concerning St. John's wort is warranted. Specifically, St. John's wort interacts with other common drugs such as: warfarin, ciclosporin, HIV protease inhibitors, selective serotonin reuptake inhibitors, and oral contraceptives thereby affecting drug metabolism. Metabolism of medications is the way in which your body breaks down ingested drugs before they can be eliminated from the body. When a drug's metabolism is inhibited, toxic levels of that drug could build up in your body in a relatively short amount of time. In addition to interacting with other drugs, the purity of many natural medicines including St. John's wort is always questionable and contaminants often lead to other undesirable effects.

So, what should you do if you suffer from SAD? First, seasonal affective disorder is a serious problem. If you believe that you may have SAD, contact your physician immediately. As mentioned previously, light therapy works in most individuals and produces virtually no side effects whereas St. John's wort interacts with other medications, which can lead to other serious problems.   Finally, some foods are thought to contain depression-fighting components.

Observational studies indicate that individuals who consume foods rich in omega-3 fatty acids are less likely to develop depression [104].   Specifically, population studies found that countries that consume more fish have less overall depression and infrequent fish consumption increases your chances of developing depression by 31% [104]. Although the ways in which omega-3 fatty acids protect against depression are not fully understood, some researchers believe that they may enhance neuronal signaling. So, what foods contain omega-3 fatty acids? Certain omega-3 fatty acids are found in walnuts, soybeans, and green, leafy vegetables while others are found in fatty fish such as salmon, mackerel, and herring.

Foods containing folic acid, a compound that may be involved in neurotransmitter (chemical messengers in the brain) synthesis or neuronal signaling, may also help fight depression [105]. Because folic acid levels may be reduced in some individuals suffering from depression, consumption of foods that are high in folic acid such as green vegetables and egg yolk may improve symptoms in depressed individuals.

From the Spice Rack to the Bedroom?

Anyone that has recently checked their e-mail or watched evening television is well aware that the advertisements for male sexual enhancers have risen through the roof in the past years with the advent of Viagra, Cialis, Levitra, etc. As with all prescription medications, potential side effects have led other researchers to hunt for natural products that aid in male sexual performance without producing unwanted side effects. After analyzing various traditional medicines that may be used for male sexual disorders, researchers uncovered nutmeg as a potential natural aphrodisiac.

Nutmeg comes from the dried seed of the *Myristica fragrans* evergreen tree and is used in a variety of dishes in French, English, Indian, West Indian, and Asian cuisines. As with many natural foods, nutmeg consumption may have certain health benefits which will be highlighted in this article. It should be mentioned here that nutmeg ingestion alone (the whole nut and not as food seasoning) is not recommended. Direct consumption of nutmeg leads to many toxic symptoms which eventually lead to hospitalization. Now, to answer the age old question, does it really work?

Along with its unique flavoring, *Myristica fragrans* may aid in the treatment or management of male sexual disorders as well as increasing libido. In Unani (Middle Eastern) traditional medicine, nutmeg is used as an aphrodisiac in cases of sexual debility and depressed desire [106]. In order to test the viability of nutmeg as an aphrodisiac, researchers administered a nutmeg extract to animals and measured many parameters associated with sexual function including mounting frequency, erection frequency, and duration of coitus [107]. In fact, animals that were treated with the nutmeg extract exhibited increased frequency of sexual encounters as well as a lengthening of time spent per sexual encounter, indicating that nutmeg may indeed prove to be a powerful aphrodisiac in humans. Although no study has addressed how nutmeg works to improve sexual function, some groups believe that it either induces changes in brain neurotransmitter (chemical messengers) levels or hormonal concentrations.

So, is nutmeg the natural answer to male sexual disorders? The short answer is we just don't know. Although nutmeg has long been used in traditional medicine, there have been no studies that address the effects of nutmeg consumption in the diet with increased sexual performance. Furthermore, while the above mentioned study does show that nutmeg extracts improve sexual performance in animals, differences in nutmeg extract preparation versus dietary consumption of nutmeg must be considered.

As mentioned previously, consumption of large amounts of nutmeg (over 20 grams or 2-3 seeds) produces many undesired, toxic symptoms such as dry mouth, nausea, anxiety, hallucinogenic delusions, and flushed skin [108]. One of the active components in nutmeg, myristicin, is believed to possess both psychotropic and hallucinogenic features, resulting in abuse and eventual overdose by drug addicts every year. Because every natural product consists of multiple compounds with potent activity, ingestion of either extracts or supplements must be done with caution. For most medicinal foods, normal (regular) dietary ingestion is sufficient to produce the desired effects.

Along with increased sexual performance, nutmeg has been used in traditional medicines for many other purposes including aiding digestion and fighting diarrhea [109,110]. Specifically, in Brazilian traditional medicine, nutmeg is one of many natural substances used for diarrhea. Subsequently, researchers studied the effect of nutmeg on rotavirus (a virus that causes gastroenteritis, fever, vomiting, stomach pain, and diarrhea that results in dehydration and in many instances death in infants and toddlers) and determined that nutmeg inhibits rotavirus propagation (spread and proliferation) [109]. Furthermore, nutmeg may also possess anti-inflammatory, anti-thrombotic, and anti-fungal properties possibly making it useful for treatment of other various infections [106].

In addition to providing a treatment for male sexual disorders and fighting infection, nutmeg may have some anti-thrombotic (prevents platelet aggregation) properties. Consequently, the potential effects of nutmeg on heart disease were analyzed in another animal model. Nutmeg decreased total cholesterol as well as LDL (bad cholesterol) and triglyceride levels [110]. Because increased cholesterol and LDL are important indicators of heart disease, the cholesterol lowering effect along with prevention of platelet aggregation may make nutmeg an important dietary means of preventing heart disease.

Does consumption of foods that contain caffeine increase your metabolism and help you lose weight?

As with food, beverages are composed of a combination of biologically active components, some of which may aid or hinder weight loss. Some of the most common caffeinated beverages include coffee, tea, soft drinks and hot chocolate. Most of the research concerning caffeine consumption and weight loss pertain to either coffee or green tea. So, this article will focus on those beverages with respect to weight loss. Because soft drinks are not recommended by the Plateau-Proof diet, they will not be considered in this article. Finally, although caffeine supplements or pills are readily available, this article is concerned with modest caffeine intake derived through beverage or chocolate consumption and not highly concentrated caffeine supplements which may pose substantial health risks.

Because caffeine is commonly known as a nervous stimulant, the creators of this dieting myth concluded that consumption of caffeine may induce weight loss by stimulating more physical activity or energy expenditure and, thus, weight loss. However, population studies find that people who drink caffeinated coffee are prone to participate in unhealthy habits such as smoking, are less physically active, and consume unhealthy diets all of which frequently lead to weight gain [111].

So, what is the effect of caffeine consumption in people trying to lose weight? Research into the usefulness of caffeine to enhance weight loss has determined that caffeine ingestion may aid in weight loss, but only slightly [112]. Caffeinated beverage consumption may stimulate energy expenditure by increasing thermogenesis (the burning of calories as heat in the body)

[102,113]. Individuals with low energy expenditure tend to have impaired appetite control, which is improved once energy expenditure increases [114]. Furthermore, caffeine consumption may decrease body fat mass since caffeine helps break down fat in adipose (fat) cells [115].

However, during the weight maintenance phase (after reaching your target weight), people who consume low levels of caffeine (around 2 cups or 150 mg/day) in the form of green tea maintained their weight better than those who consumed caffeine alone or high amounts of caffeine via green tea (around 550 mg/day) [112]. In fact, caffeine-induced thermogenesis is more likely to occur in lean versus obese individuals, indicating that caffeinated beverage consumption is more likely to aid in weight maintenance as opposed to weight loss [116].

Because people who consumed similar amounts of caffeine alone (in the form of a caffeine supplement) did not maintain their weight loss, this indicates that other components in teas and coffees may aid in weight loss maintenance. For example, along with caffeine, coffee also contains potassium, niacin, magnesium, antioxidants and chlorogenic acid all of which may participate in maintenance of weight reduction [117].

Moderate consumption of caffeine (less than 300 mg/day, equivalent to 3 cups of coffee) is not associated with adverse effects like general toxicity, cardiovascular effects, bone status, calcium balance, change in adult behavior, cancer or male fertility [118]. However, it is advised that women of reproductive age partially limit caffeine intake to about 200 mg/day. Finally, children should consume far less caffeine (less than 100 mg/day).

As with food items, beverages are also classified in the CP and FP tables in the Plateau-Proof Diet. Depending on which specialized Plateau-Proof Diet you are using, be sure to verify if your favorite caffeine-containing beverage is found in the green tables for each rotation.

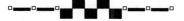

Cereals - Not Just for Breakfast

After the U.S. Congress passed the Nutrition Labeling and Education Act in 1990, the Food and Drug Administration made its first health claim pertaining to a specific food in 1999, announcing that 'Diets rich in whole grain foods and other plant foods and low in total fat, saturated fat, and cholesterol may reduce the risk of heart disease and some cancers'. Because the average American consumes less than 1 serving of whole grains per day, other dietary guidelines include 'Eat plenty of cereal foods, preferably whole grain and without added fat, salt, or sugar'.

Almost forty years ago, epidemiological evidence suggested that people who eat more cereal were less likely to develop heart disease. Subsequent studies confirmed that cereal consumption decreases total cholesterol and LDL cholesterol levels. There is a link between cholesterol levels and heart disease. In fact, an individual's risk of developing heart disease increases 4 times when their cholesterol levels rise to 264 mg/dl as compared to the normal levels of 167 mg/dl [119]. Furthermore, slight reductions in cholesterol levels by 1% reduce heart disease mortality by 2% [119].

Cereals, particularly whole grains are high in dietary fiber. Dietary fiber are carbohydrates from plants that humans cannot digest. We cannot digest fiber because we don't have the enzymes in our small intestines that are required to break it down. Consequently, we cannot absorb dietary fiber into our bodies. Furthermore, fibers can be divided into soluble and insoluble with soluble fiber possessing lipid lowering activities. Examples of soluble fiber are pectins, gums, and mucilages all of which possess gel forming properties. Increased soluble fiber consumption lowers total cholesterol and LDL cholesterol levels [120]. Particularly, oats are high in Beta-glucan, a soluble nonstarch fiber. Although the exact mechanism by which fiber consumption lowers your risk of developing heart disease is currently not known, some evidence indicates that fiber may interfere with absorption of dietary fats or inhibit cholesterol production [119].

Cereals are made up of polyunsaturated fats, fiber, vitamin E, selenium, and folic acid. Vitamin E and selenium are both potent antioxidants, and consumption of antioxidants reduces the risk of developing heart disease. Finally, folic acid reduces plasma homocysteine levels which may be connected to heart disease progression [121].

Categories of cereal foods that may lower your risk of developing CHD include cereals such as wheat, rice, maize, barley, oats, and rye. Importantly, the health benefits derived from cereals are specifically with respect to whole grains and not processed or refined grains. Because the refining process removes the bran from the grains, refining essentially removes at least half of the fiber derived from the grain. Furthermore, during the refining process, 90% of the selenium, 80% of the vitamin E, and 25% of the protein is lost [120].

Along with adding a pleasant nutty flavor to your morning breakfast or baked good, oat consumption lowers total cholesterol and LDL (bad cholesterol) levels, thereby reducing the risk of heart disease. Additionally, rice bran and barley also lowered blood cholesterol levels although to a smaller extent. This is most likely due to the fact that most individuals typically consume polished, white rice that has been refined and very rarely consume barley. However, wheat fiber, which is primarily composed of insoluble fiber, doesn't appear to possess lipid lowering activities [120].

So, how much fiber should a person consume to derive any health benefits? Consuming 10 grams of fiber per day is associated with decreasing your risk of developing heart disease by 14% and reducing your risk of coronary mortality by 27% [122]. As a reference, 3 grams of fiber is approximately equivalent to 1-½ cups of oats and it is recommended that the average person consume more than 3 servings of whole grains/day [123].

Finally, consumption of whole grains may benefit individuals with Type II diabetes. Observational studies indicate that people who consume more fiber are less likely to be overweight and develop insulin resistance [122,124]. Because whole grains take more time for your body to digest, they typically don't produce significant rises in blood glucose [124]. Fiber consumption may help stabilize blood glucose levels since changing from a low fiber to high fiber diet resulted in a reduction in blood glucose levels by 10% [124]. Furthermore, this observation was more evident in overweight individuals who are more at risk for developing Type II diabetes.

Is Cinnamon the God Spice for Type II Diabetics?

The incidence of Type II diabetes is on the rise in the United States, and it is directly related to the obesity epidemic currently occurring in the U.S. This portion will discuss the benefits of dietary consumption of cinnamon on stabilizing blood glucose levels in persons with Type II diabetes. However, replacing any current medication with cinnamon or suspending the use of any medication is not recommended. Individuals with Type II diabetes should consult their physician before making any dietary changes.

Given the side effects from drugs commonly used to combat Type II diabetes, the search for dietary means to stabilize blood glucose levels in Type II diabetes is a constant quest. For example, some of the potential side effects include: weight gain, upset stomach, rash, nausea, weakness, dizziness, anemia, and liver diseases. One class of drugs used for Type II diabetes, sulfonylureas, induces increased insulin secretion by the pancreas as well as aid in glucose clearance from the blood. However, because of the numerous side effects such as low blood sugar, blurred vision, cold sweats, headache, nausea, and weakness as well as others, associated with sulfonylureas, alternative food-based, dietary means of stabilizing blood glucose in individuals with Type II diabetes would be highly beneficial[125].

Cinnamon, derived from the inner bark of *Cinnamonum cassia, Cinnamonum saigonicum,* or *Cinnamonum zeylanicum* as well as leaves in the form of oil, has long been used by people in Korea, China, and Russia suffering from Type II diabetes. There are a number of ways in which cinnamon consumption is thought to affect Type II diabetes, including increasing insulin sensitivity by increasing plasma insulin levels and possibly by mimicking insulin itself[126,127].

A key study performed by Khan *et al.* addressed the potential use of cinnamon as a treatment for Type II diabetes[128]. The individuals recruited for this test were diagnosed with Type II diabetes, over the age of 40, and currently not taking insulin. Furthermore, their fasting blood glucose was between 140-400 mg/dl. At the beginning of the study, blood glucose, triglyceride, and serum cholesterol levels were measured for each participant. Then, study participants received capsules containing either cinnamon derived from *Cinnamonum cassia* or wheat flour (placebo controls) and were instructed to take 1, 3, or 6 grams each day for 40 days. Again blood glucose, triglyceride, and serum cholesterol levels were measured after 20 days and 40 days in addition to 20 days after the participants ceased taking the capsules. This study showed that cinnamon consumption in any amount for 20 or 40 days decreased blood glucose levels 18-30% as well as triglycerides and serum cholesterol (13-26%). Importantly, LDL (bad cholesterol) was reduced by 10-24% in participants consuming cinnamon while HDL (good cholesterol) was unaffected.

In order to determine the long term effects of cinnamon intake on stabilizing blood glucose and serum cholesterol levels, final measurements were taken 20 days after finishing the cinnamon capsules. Interestingly, blood glucose levels remained lowered 20 days after the cinnamon treatment. Furthermore, lowered serum triglycerides, cholesterol, and LDL were observed in participants that consumed the cinnamon 20 days later. Because the beneficial effects of cinnamon were sustained long after its consumption, it may not be necessary to consume cinnamon daily to receive its benefits. Importantly, subjects that took the wheat flour capsules did not have any change in blood glucose or lipid profiles, indicating that the beneficial effects obtained from the cinnamon capsules is specific. The one drawback from this study is that there were relatively few participants involved (60 people) and the study time was relatively short.

A follow up study indicated that not all cinnamon extracts are created equal in stabilizing blood glucose levels in Type II diabetes[127]. Specifically, *Cinnamonum cassia* was more effective than *Cinnamonum zeylanicum* at increasing insulin levels in the blood and thereby decreasing blood glucose levels. Furthermore, *Cinnamonum cassia* was almost as effective at decreasing blood glucose as glibenclamide, a commonly prescribed sulfonylurea used in the treatment for Type II diabetes.

Along with improving blood glucose and lipid profiles, cinnamon intake may also have additional benefits. Because cinnamon is high in flavinoids, it may also function as an antioxidant[129]. Antioxidants possess anti-carcinogenic characteristics as well as decrease a person's risk for developing heart disease. Furthermore, there is some evidence that cinnamon may have some antibacterial, antidermatophyte, vasodilative, as well as anti-thrombotic activities, indicating that cinnamon may also be useful in wound healing and cardioprotection[130,131].

Relatively small amounts of cinnamon (approximately ½ tsp) were sufficient to reduce both blood glucose as well as lipid levels. So, it is not necessary to purchase and consume cinnamon pills which are commercially available. Regular seasoning of meals is sufficient to receive the hypoglycemic effects of cinnamon.

The efficacy of cinnamon is controlling type II diabetes is another indication of the potency of certain medicinal foods in preventing and/or treating certain diseases, including obesity and its complications. Proper use of medicinal foods with the plateau-proof diet or the plateau-proof diet cardio may greatly improve your health while you cruise to a complete and sustainable weight loss.

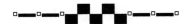

Medicinal foods and health management foods

Medicinal foods are those foods that when eaten in adequate amounts may cure a disease or relieve the symptoms of a disease. They are also foods that when eaten regularly protect the body from diseases. These foods will keep you healthy either by fighting diseases that you already have, or by protecting you from diseases that you could potentially have. The medicinal foods listed in this chapter are not limited to those that address health problems that are related to obesity. Medicinal foods that fight a broad range of diseases are included in this chapter in keeping with the clinique science weight loss philosophy – a complete weight loss that is accompanied by improved health and well being. When your body is in general good health it becomes a relatively easier task to lose weight. This is why our approach to weight loss involves getting healthier from day one. The medicinal foods listed in this chapter have all been shown to have medicinal benefits using modern scientific techniques. Along with the right types of proteins discussed in the plateau-proof diet section, these medicinal foods should form the core of your diet – that is, include them in every meal if possible.

Most of the medicinal foods listed here are herbs and spices. Although there are other plant medicines, they are not included here because they are not natural human foods. Also, I do not endorse the use of animals and/or animal parts for medicinal purposes; hence they are not included here.

Please pay very close attention, because successfully gaining good health and weight loss from medicinal foods depends greatly on using them properly. The active component of these herbs and spices usually dissolve well in oil but not as well in water. To get the most benefit from these herbs and spices, it is necessary to make oil infusions with them. Olive oil is the best to use, but you can also use other vegetable oils that have NO saturated fats and trans fats. Your choice of oil should contain monounsaturated fats and/or polyunsaturated fats only. Use dried spices and herbs whenever possible, as opposed to fresh ones. Always grind or chop them as finely as possible prior to adding them in oil. Add anywhere from three to six times the volume of oil to the volume of ground herbs and/or spices, and shake vigorously to mix well. Pour the mixture in the pan and heat briefly, without bringing the oil to a boil. [If you are using fresh herbs and spices, heat the oil while stirring until steam stops rising from the oil.] Allow the oil to cool to room temperature, then pour the oil with herbs and/or spices in an appropriate container and store it in a cool place. Combine herbs and spices creatively to make tasty and healthy infusions that address your personal health and gustatory needs. Add these infusions to everything you eat if possible – it is your ticket to a healthy weight loss.

Please be reminded that it is very important to use oil to extract the medicinal properties of these herbs and spices as described above. You may enjoy the great tastes and flavors of some of these herbs and spices in a water base, such as in soups, without getting any of the medicinal benefits. The compounds in these foods that are responsible for their tastes and flavors are not necessarily those that are responsible for their medicinal properties.

Ok – now that you know how to prepare these herbs and spices for maximum benefit, let's take a look at them. Since some herbs and spices look alike but are not equally effective medicinally, pictures and scientific names of these medicinal herbs and spices have been included below to avoid confusion. Remember to make creative combinations of these herbs and spices and to give a healthy dash to everything you eat if possible. At the end of the list I will include my special weight loss recipe which showed very good results in a limited clinical trial. This recipe hasn't been published anywhere or disclosed to anyone until now – please enjoy.

Allspice (*Pimenta dioica*)

Allspice is the fruit of the evergreen tree, *Pimenta dioica*. These small berries are harvested and sun-dried, and then off to the supermarket they go. [Actually, I prefer to buy my spices online nowadays because of the bargains. If the fancy packaging means nothing to you, you could get a large Ziploc bag full for a fraction of the price of a small, fancy bottle.] Allspice is used in a variety of curries and jerk sauces in the Caribbean, Mexico, India, and North America. If you don't know how to cook curries and jerk sauces, no problem. Simply give it a go in that leftover no-name sauce or soup you made yesterday. With its pleasant aroma suggestive of both cinnamon and clove, it is likely to excite your taste buds while keeping your body healthy. Also, with its high level of antioxidants, allspice may help you prevent cancer and heart disease, as well as help you age a little more gracefully – hmmm! Isn't that a nice reward for eating something that is delicious to begin with? There's even more to allspice. It may also lower your blood glucose levels, so if you are diabetic or are flirting with high blood glucose levels, you may find that allspice is a keeper.

Anise (*Pimpinella anisum*)

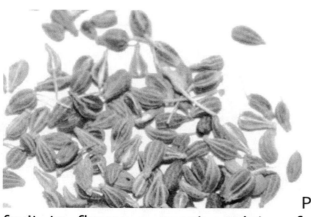

People use this licorice-flavored fruit to flavor a great variety of dishes from cookies to stew. Anise however packs more than a great flavor. Ask anyone who already stocks this beauty in their kitchen and they are likely to brag of the health benefits that they have been enjoying from it. If the bragger is a man, his high-pitch voice is likely from the estrogenic compounds in anise. Yes, anise is rich in these estrogenic compounds which are known to induce lactation, promote menstruation, ease childbirth, and increase libido – hopefully not all at the same time for you. It is clearly a must-have food when menopause starts peeping, or even when it already has you in its hold.

Anise also contains an ingredient called anethol that has anti-inflammatory and antioxidant properties. Inflammation is not as bad when there is anise in your kitchen then, is it? It is also good to know that this simple spice may help you stay cancer-free owing to its antioxidant properties. Jim, you may want to look for your antioxidants elsewhere though.

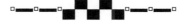

Basil *(Ocimum basilicum)*

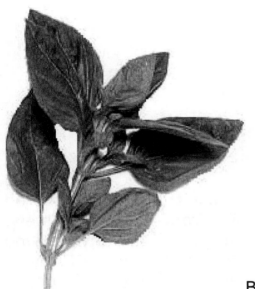

Basil (sweet basil) is the leaves of the herb *Ocimum basilicum.* This piercingly fragrant herb is common around the world, and is deservingly used to flavor a great variety of dishes worldwide. Outside of its great flavor, basil contains anti-bacterial, anti-fungal, and anti-viral properties. It is used in Chinese traditional medicine and other naturopathic medicines to prevent or cure infections.

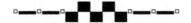

Bay Leaves (*Laurus nobilis*)

These dried leaves don't look like much, but make sure to create space for them in your spice rack. Mediterranean, French, Moroccan, and Turkish cuisines use bay leaves in soups, stews, pickles, tomato, and meat dishes. Along with providing an olfactory pleaser to your everyday dishes, they may help to increase your glucose metabolism, thus lowering your blood glucose levels. This is obviously beneficial to diabetics, but also to overweight people who don't yet have problems with hyperglycemia.

Black Pepper (*Piper nigrum*)

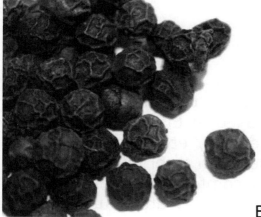

Black and White Pepper are both the dried berries of *Piper nigrum*. To produce black pepper, the berries are picked while still green. Black pepper is used around the world in spice blends such as salad dressings and other infusions. In addition to adding flavor to food, black pepper is commonly used in Ayurvedic medicine (an ancient form of Indian medicine) and thought to balance the various constituents of blood. Specifically, black pepper consumption helps to reduce total blood cholesterol levels, decreasing LDL (bad cholesterol) and increasing HDL (good cholesterol) in people with high blood cholesterol levels. Additionally, it also helps to reduce blood triglyceride levels. Thus, black pepper consumption may decrease the risk of developing heart disease by decreasing both cholesterol levels as well as oxidative stress in individuals at risk for heart disease.

Caraway Seed (*Carum carvi*)

Caraway is the dried fruit of the herb *Carum carvi*. It is commonly used in Europe to flavor rye bread, biscuits, carrot and potato dishes, etc. I hope you like their flavor because you can also use them to prevent or to treat your dyspepsia (stomach pain or discomfort including bloating, heart burn, upset stomach, and belching). Watch out though if you have problems with portion control – it stimulates the appetite.

Cardamom (*Elettaria cardamomum*)

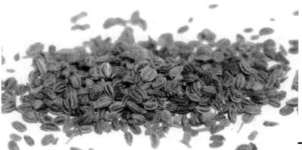

Cardamom is the dried fruit of the perennial *Elettaria cardamomum.* It is commonly used in Asian, North African, and Middle Eastern cuisines. Its medicinal benefits include the treatment of gastrointestinal disorders such as gastritis (inflammation of the stomach lining) and peptic ulcers. It has also been shown to be effective for the treatment of gastric lesions induced by alcohol.

Celery seed (*Apium graveolens*)

This relative of the vegetable celery is commonly used in German, Italian, and Russian cuisines for pickling, salad dressings, and soups. In addition to their gustatory allure, celery seeds are used as a treatment for many conditions including low libido, gas, and rheumatoid arthritis. I stock these seeds in my spice rack because of their high antioxidant content. They are valuable for good cardiovascular health as well as for cancer prevention. They also contain a compound called apigenin which may slow down or inhibit the progression of liver cancer. Make space in your spice rack for this one.

Chervil (*Anthriscus cerefolium*)

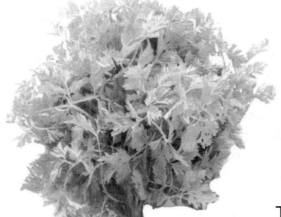

These leaves of the fern-like plant *Anthriscus cerefolium* will give mouth-watering character to your poultry, fish, and soups. In many traditional medicines, chervil leaves have been used to treat circulatory disorders, while the root has been used to treat anemia in Japan and China. Chervil leaves have a high free radical scavenging activity as well as antioxidant activity. Chervil may therefore prevent cardiovascular disease by helping the body get rid of dangerous free radicals and by preventing the oxidation of lipids - a key step in the progression of heart disease.

Cinnamon (*Cinnamomum cassia*)

Cinnamon is derived from the dried inner bark of members of the *Cinnamomum* evergreen tree family. In addition to being used in a majority of baked goods, cinnamon is also used in a variety of other dishes such as curries and moles. If your palette is set like mine, then this royal spice has tickled your nose and tormented you with a richness of nature's delight. Yes, don't hesitate to smack your lips for this one, especially if you are suffering from Type II diabetes or if you are hyperglycemic. Cinnamon has long been used in traditional medicine for treating Type II diabetes. It may alleviate the symptoms of Type II diabetes in a number of ways, including; increasing insulin sensitivity, increasing plasma insulin levels, and possibly mimicking insulin itself. Furthermore, there is some evidence that cinnamon may have some antibacterial, antidermatophyte, vasodilative, as well as anti-thrombotic activities. In other words stock it in your kitchen and stuff yourself with it for good cardiovascular health, or if you have problems with wound healing.

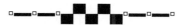

Clove (*Syzygium aromaticum*)

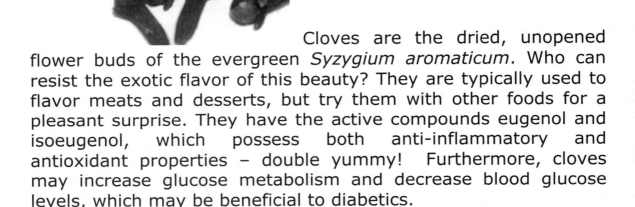

Cloves are the dried, unopened flower buds of the evergreen *Syzygium aromaticum*. Who can resist the exotic flavor of this beauty? They are typically used to flavor meats and desserts, but try them with other foods for a pleasant surprise. They have the active compounds eugenol and isoeugenol, which possess both anti-inflammatory and antioxidant properties – double yummy! Furthermore, cloves may increase glucose metabolism and decrease blood glucose levels, which may be beneficial to diabetics.

Cocoa [very dark] (*Theobroma cacao*)

Very dark cocoa (drinking chocolate) is a sinfully tasty treat. Amazingly, this beauty can directly cause weight loss by disrupting the storage of fat in fat cells. It also can cause weight loss by increasing the burn rate of glucose and fat in your body, in a process called diet-induced thermogenesis. You have to be very careful that you stock your kitchen with the very dark stuff (70% or more cocoa).The dark cocoa should be sugar-free. Add it to hot water or to hot milk (fat-free) according to manufacturer's directions or to your taste. Enjoy!

Caution! Drinking the wrong type of cocoa may result in weight gain.

Coriander *(Coriandum sativum)*

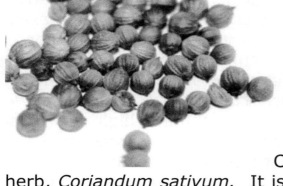

Coriander is the dried fruit of the herb, *Coriandum sativum.* It is used in a great variety of dishes around the world, but most commonly in stews, curries, and lentils. The value of a little dash of coriander is more than marginal, both in taste and in health benefits. It is used in traditional medicine to relieve dyspepsia (stomach pain or discomfort including bloating, heart burn, upset stomach, and belching), anxiety, and insomnia.

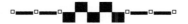

Cumin (*Cuminum cyminum*)

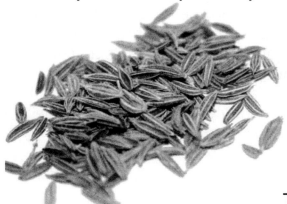

These dried seeds of the herb *Cuminum cyminum* should have a permanent place in your spice rack. It is sold by itself or in spice blends such as garam masala and curry powder. Let your taste drive your pick. It is common is some Mexican, Indian, and Thai cuisines, and you certainly should make this gift of nature common in your home cuisine too. Past that incredible flavor, cumin may deliver some significant good to your health. It contains high levels of antioxidants, suggesting that it may be helpful in reducing the risk of cancer and heart disease. It also possesses hypoglycemic activity, lowering blood glucose levels. In traditional Ayurvedic medicine (an ancient form of Indian medicine), cumin has long been used as a remedy for diarrhea, flatulence, and indigestion. It seems like a little cumin after a bean meal is not a bad idea.

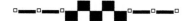

Dillweed (*Anethum graveolens*)

Dillweed is commonly used in dill pickles as well as in potato and meat dishes. In traditional folk medicine, dill is used as a treatment for gastrointestinal illnesses such as stomach ache, flatulence, and indigestion.

Fennel (*Foeniculum vulgare*)

The dried fruit of *Foeniculum vulgare*, fennel is used to flavor fish, meats, and even baked goods. Like anise, fennel has estrogenic compounds that can induce milk secretion, promote menstruation, increase libido, and ease childbirth. An active compound in fennel, anethol, has both anti-oxidant and anti-inflammatory activities, suggesting that it may block inflammation and help prevent cancer. The estrogen-like compounds in fennel make it beneficial for relieving menopausal symptoms, including the prevention of post-menopausal bone loss.

Fenugreek (*Trigonella foenum-graecum*)

Fenugreek spice is the dried seeds of *Trigonella foenum-graecum*. It is most common in Indian and Middle Eastern cuisines. You may have had it in a curry or in mango chutney, if it isn't already in your spice rack. It is a component of curry powder. Egyptian folk medicine uses fenugreek to lower blood sugar levels in diabetics. Fenugreek may also inhibit weight gain that is induced by a high fat diet.

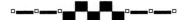

Garlic [fresh bulb] (*Allium sativum*)

Garlic is common worldwide, but many people do not know of its health benefits. It can be used to flavor most vegetable, fish, and meat dishes. In traditional medicines, garlic is used in the treatment of gastrointestinal disorders. An active component of garlic, diallyl sulfide, may prevent the formation of new tumors, particularly gastric and colorectal cancers. Garlic also reduces serum cholesterol, blood pressure, and blood clotting, thus reducing the risk of heart disease. Please note that these benefits are not observed with the consumption of garlic powder. To get these benefits you should use unprocessed bulbs of garlic. Some people use garlic supplements – a topic discussed elsewhere in this book.

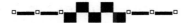

Ginger (*Zingiber officinale*)

Ginger is the root of the herb *Zingiber officinale.* Although ginger is common in many spice blends from India, China and Europe, try using it pure to give a mesmerizing flavor to whatever is brewing in your kitchen today. You didn't know that it is good for weight loss did you? Yes it is.

Alone, ginger has a relatively week potential to stimulate weight loss. When it is combined with the leaves of chickweed (my secret formula) and brewed as a herbal tea, this combination becomes a potent stimulator of weight loss. I discovered this combination almost serendipitously in the late 90s. A limited clinical study a few years later confirmed the potency of this combination, with an average weight loss of about 4 lbs per week. I will discuss this combination in detail a little later.

Ginger has additional therapeutic uses. Traditional Chinese medicine uses it to treat nausea. It works very well for treating a cough too – just bite and chew a small piece and repeat until the cough vanishes (usually within 5 to 10 minutes). An active compound in ginger, gingerol, possesses anti-thrombotic activity, making it possibly useful in the prevention of heart disease.

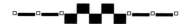

Mace (*Myristica fragrans*)

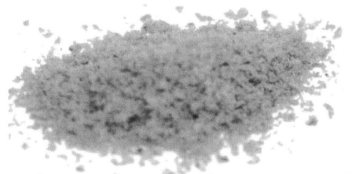

Mace is the thin shell that surrounds nutmeg, the fruit of the *Myristica fragrans* tree. Mace is used in a variety of dishes in French, English, Indian, West Indian, and Asian cuisines. Along with its delicate flavoring, *Myristica fragrans* may aid in the treatment or management of male sexual disorders, including libido enhancement. It also appears to possess anti-inflammatory, anti-diarrheal, anti-thrombotic and anti-fungal properties.

Nutmeg (*Myristica fragrans*)

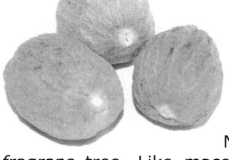

Nutmeg is the fruit of the *Myristica fragrans* tree. Like mace, it is used in a variety of dishes in French, English, Indian, West Indian, and Asian cuisines. It has a warm inviting flavor that reminds me dotingly of the baking lessons I took in my mother's kitchen as a boy. Like mace, it may also be used in the treatment or management of male sexual disorders - libido problems included. It also appears to possess anti-inflammatory, anti-diarrheal, anti-thrombotic and anti-fungal properties.

Oregano (*Origanum vulgare)*

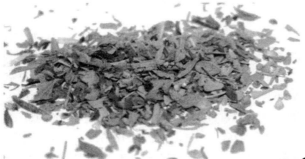

Oregano is derived from the dried leaves of the herb *Origanum vulgare*. Oregano is widely used in flavoring tomato, meat, and soup dishes in North America and the Mediterranean. You probably already know that a good dash of this beauty makes your food twice as fun – especially if you keep the dish simple. This is super, healthy fun since oregano contains high levels of antioxidants that may help you prevent cancer and heart disease, as well as slow the wheels of aging a little. In addition, oregano may help stabilize blood glucose levels in diabetics – bang!

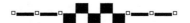

Paprika (*Capsicum annum*)

Paprika is made from the ground pods of *Capsicum annum* sweet, red pepper plant. Remember that flavor that makes you crave a bowl of chili? It can also be used to flavor a great variety of dishes – add a little or a bunch as dictated by your taste buds – you can't go wrong here. Paprika and hot peppers have a compound called capsaicin that may contribute to weight loss. It contains high levels of antioxidants, suggesting that they may be helpful in the prevention of cancer, heart disease and ungraceful aging. It also has antimicrobial activity – may be helpful the next time food poisoning ties you down. Capsaicin is also effective for pain management. It is the component of peppers that make it hot. Hotter peppers such as jalopeño and habanero would therefore be expected to be more potent than the sweet red pepper from which paprika is made.

Parsley (*Petroselinum crispum*)

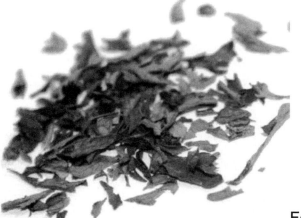

Forget about just using these leaves of the herb, *Petroselinum crispum* as garnish. You want to chow down on this beauty. Throw in generous amounts in your stews, soups, and sauces, because excessive consumption of parsley may help you lose weight. Nice, isn't it? Parsley is also known to help enhance memory and to help stabilize blood glucose levels in diabetics. Nice!

Poppy seeds (*Papaver somniferum*)

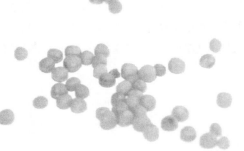

Poppy seeds come from the dried seeds of the annual *Papaver somniferum.* Poppy seeds are used in breads, rolls and salad dressings in many countries. In India and Turkey, crushed poppy seeds are used in various spice mixtures. Crushed poppy seeds in a spice mixture may be used for pain management. It also is used in naturopathic medicine as a cough suppressant.

Red/Cayenne Pepper (*Capsicum frutescens*)

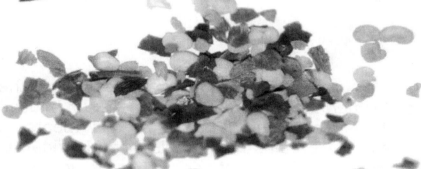

Red pepper is the dried fruit of *Capsicum frutescens.* It is used in a variety of foods including meats, seafood, and pickles in Indian, Mexican, and Caribbean cuisines. In addition to adding a spicy flavor to your favorite dishes, it may provide some beneficial therapeutic effects. It is used to treat diabetes in Jamaican folk medicine. The active component of red pepper, capsaicin, stimulates insulin release and contributes in stabilizing blood glucose levels. In Mayan traditional medicine, red pepper was used as a treatment for infected wounds and fresh burns (ouch!). It has been scientifically shown to possess antimicrobial activity.

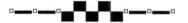

Rosemary (*Rosmarinus officinalis*)

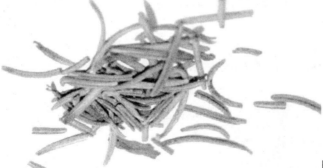

Rosemary comes from the dried leaves of the *Rosmarinus officinalis* evergreen. It is used as a garnish as well as seasoning for the various meats in Mediterranean cuisines. It contains high levels of anti-oxidants, and is believed to protect against heptotoxicity (liver toxicity). It is also used in naturopathic medicine to treat asthma, eczema, and rheumatism.

Saffron (*Crocus sativus*)

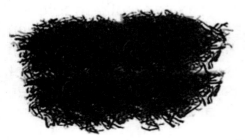

Saffron is derived from the dried flowers of the *Crocus sativus.* Saffron adds a rich yellow color and inviting flavor to cheeses, rice, and seafood. It is rich in anti-oxidants, which aid in wound healing and cancer prevention, as well as contribute to a more graceful aging. In Persian traditional medicine, saffron is used to treat anxiety and depression. It is used in other naturopathic medicine to treat stomach disorders, as a digestive aid, and in appetite stimulation. The appetite stimulation part is contradictory to conventional weight loss techniques that employ appetite suppression. If you think you may have problems with portion control, and believe that some or all of your weight problems is from overeating, saffron may not be a good choice of medicinal food for you.

Sage (*Salvia officinalis)*

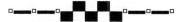Sage comes from the dried leaves of the herb, *Salvia officinalis*. It is commonly used to flavor fish, poultry, and sausages. In Iranian traditional medicine, sage is used as a treatment for diabetes due to its hypoglycemic activity. Furthermore, sage also possesses anti-bacterial, anti-fungal, and anti-viral activities.

Savory (*Satureja hortensis*)

Savory is derived from the leaves of the herb, *Satureja hortensis.* In the Mediterranean region, savory is used in vegetable, bean, egg, and soup dishes. Don't worry – you don't have to call the Mediterranean for it. There is enough of it waiting for you at your local spice market, and even more options (less expensive) online, if you shop as "smartly" as I do.

Savory is used in Iranian traditional medicine to treat stomach and intestinal disorders such as cramps, nausea, and diarrhea. It also possesses anti-bacterial properties, making it a possible remedy for gastroenteritis as well as infectious diarrhea.

Sesame seed (*Sesamum indicum*)

Sesame seeds come from the herb *Sesamum indicum*. They are typically used in breads and rolls, and as seasoning in Middle Eastern and Asian cuisines. These seeds are rich in antioxidants, suggesting that they may be helpful in the prevention of cancer and heart disease. Of course, the antioxidants also slow down the aging process a little.

Tarragon (*Artemisia dracunculus*)

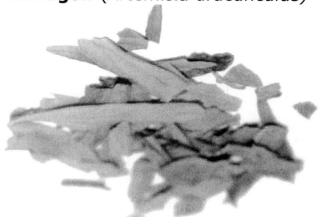

Tarragon is derived from the dried leaves of the herb, *Artemisia dracunculus.* It is used in a variety of sauces, most commonly in French cuisine. In Iranian traditional medicine, it is used as a treatment for anxiety and epilepsy. It is rich in antioxidants and therefore has the potential to help prevent cancer and heart disease, as well as to contribute to a more graceful aging. It also possesses antifungal activity – in case you find yourself in that bind.

Thyme (*Thymus vulgaris*)

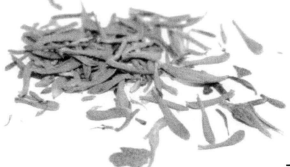

Thyme is derived from the dried leaves of the perennial, *Thymus vulgaris.* It is typically used to flavor meats, fish, stews, and stuffings. Along with its alluring flavor, thyme possesses anti-thrombotic (anti-clotting) activities, and is potentially useful in the prevention of heart disease.

Turmeric (*Curcuma longa*)

Turmeric comes from the root of *Curcuma longa*. It adds a characteristic bright yellow color to any dish, and is typically used to flavor mustard, relish, chutneys, and rice dishes in the Caribbean, India, North Africa, Middle East and Indonesia. In Ayurvedic (an ancient form of Indian medicine) traditional medicine, it is used as an anti-inflammatory agent. Additionally, because the active component of turmeric, curcumin, decreases blood cholesterol, turmeric consumption may reduce the risk of heart disease. Finally, turmeric consumption may improve Crohn's disease, psoriasis, Alzheimer's disease and other adult dementias.

White Pepper (*Piper nigrum*)

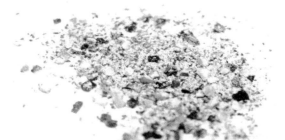

Black and White Pepper are both derived from the dried berry of *Piper nigrum*. To produce white pepper, the berries are picked when fully ripe. It is typically used to flavor sauces and soups. It is used in traditional medicine to balance various constituents of blood. Specifically, it decreases blood LDL cholesterol (bad cholesterol) and triglyceride levels, and increases HDL cholesterol (good cholesterol) levels. It may decrease the risk of developing heart disease by balancing cholesterol levels and by reducing oxidative stress.

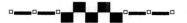

My special weight loss formula

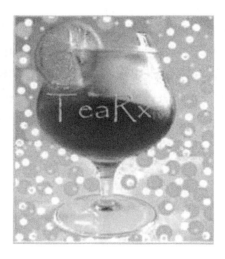

After several years of studying medicinal plants and experimenting with them in lab, I found a simple combination that makes a difference in weight loss. I have not published this anywhere, and I have not disclosed this formula until now. Chickweed (*Stellaria media*) is a plant (vegetable) that has very little effect on weight loss when it is consumed alone. Ginger (*Zingiber officinale*) also has little or no effect on weight loss when it is consumed alone. When chickweed is combined with ginger in a tea formulation, they become a potent facilitator of weight loss.

How to make the tea formulation:

- Combine 3 volumes of dried chickweed aerial parts (stems and leaves) with one volume of fresh ginger, e.g. 3 cups of chickweed to 1 cup of ginger.

- Add the mixture into a blender or food processor and blend together to form a reasonably homogenous mixture.
- Add 16 volumes of water (e.g. 3 cups of chickweed, 1 cup of ginger and 16 cups of water) and mix to form a reasonably homogenous mixture.
- Add the mixture to a tea pot or other type of pot and heat to a boil.
- [OPTIONAL] Add ½ a cup of rum or another 80 proof (40% alcohol) drink as determined by your taste and mix well.
- Strain the tea into a tea cup and enjoy it hot or chill it and enjoy it on the rocks. Use sugar-free sweetener if you would like to sweeten it.

Please note that I am not claiming that this is a magical weight loss potion. You still will have to follow the advice and directives in this book to enjoy a complete weight loss and improved health. This formulation will simply help in making you lose weight faster. It is important that you talk with your doctor before using this formulation, just like with any other information in this book. Although these are natural foods different people may have different reactions to them, some of which may be undesirable. The weight loss formulation that I have presented above is for information purposes only, and is in no way intended to constitute a treatment or cure for obesity.

Caution!
Don't attempt to increase the rate of your weight loss by substituting meals for this herbal tea. Don't drink more than 3 pints of this herbal tea per day.

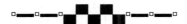

The health management foods

Health management foods are not as potent in their therapeutic properties as the medicinal foods described above. They however will actively contribute to prevent disease when they are integrated into a healthy diet. Some of these foods can also help to alleviate a disease condition when they are integrated into a healthy diet with the appropriate medicinal foods. These foods should be eaten in the appropriate rotation of the plateau-proof diet or the plateau-proof diet cardio as applicable (see chapters 4 & 5). Here is a list of common health management foods and their putative benefits:

Apple: May help lower bad cholesterol levels. It may also help to reduce the risk for cancer. It may promote regularity, and may also help control appetite.

Asparagus: Helps promote regularity due to its high fiber content. It may also contribute to cancer prevention due to its high antioxidant content.

Avocado: May maintain or enhance cardiovascular health by decreasing the concentration of bad cholesterol in the blood. It is also rich in antioxidants that are beneficial in cancer prevention.

Banana: May help to relieve an upset stomach. It may also help replenish body potassium levels, which is beneficial during rigorous exercise.

Barley: May enhance cardiovascular health by decreasing the concentration of bad cholesterol in the blood. It is also rich in antioxidants, and thus is beneficial in cancer prevention. It is also capable of killing some of the viruses that infect us.

Beans: These are excellent foods for lowering the concentration of bad cholesterol in blood. All types of beans – black, kidney, navy, pinto, etc and other legumes such as soy beans and lentils fall in this category. They are also high in fiber and protein, making them an excellent food source for people who want to lose weight. The same properties also make them an excellent food source for people with diabetes or the metabolic syndrome. Beans may also contribute to the prevention of certain cancers. It is a very important food for maintaining and improving health. Beans may have a mild adverse effect in some people that is readily reversible with over-the-counter anti-gas medications.

Beets: May be helpful in relieving malaise. They are rich in iron, and therefore may prevent or relieve certain types of anemia. They may also have some anti-inflammatory properties, as they have been shown to be beneficial for conditions such as acne and gout. Beets are also a good food source for people who are trying to lose weight. Due to its high iron content, people suffering from type-II diabetes should avoid beets.

Bell Pepper: May contribute to the prevention of certain cancers due to their antioxidant content.

Blueberry: Has some anti-bacterial and anti-viral activity. May also help relieve diarrhea.

Broccoli: When broccoli is only slightly cooked or eaten raw, it is rich in antioxidants that are known to contribute to the prevention of several types of cancers. It may lower the risk of breast cancer by controlling blood estrogen levels. It is rich in fiber, and is a cholesterol lowering food. It is a good food for people who are trying to lose weight. It is also a good food for people with high blood cholesterol levels and for people with type-II diabetes.

Brussels sprouts: Just like broccoli, when Brussels sprouts are only slightly cooked or eaten raw, they are rich in antioxidants that are known to contribute to the prevention of several types of cancers. They may also lower the risk of breast cancer by controlling blood estrogen levels.

Cabbage: Rich in antioxidants and is a potent contributor to the prevention of several types of cancers. It is known to lower blood estrogen levels, and to contribute in the prevention of breast cancer. As is the case with other vegetables, prolonged cooking reduces the potency of cabbage. It is ideal to eat it raw or slightly cooked.

Carrot: Rich in a potent antioxidant called beta carotene. Beta carotene from carrots may contribute to the prevention of certain types of cancers. It may also improve cardiovascular health, as well as improve the body's ability to fight infections. Carrots are good for the eyes too. Regular consumption of carrots could contribute to the lowering of blood cholesterol levels.

Cauliflower: Like broccoli, Brussels sprouts and cabbage, when cauliflower is only slightly cooked or eaten raw, it is rich in antioxidants that are known to contribute to the prevention of several types of cancers. They may also lower the risk of breast cancer by controlling blood estrogen levels.

Celery: May help in the prevention of certain cancers due to its content of antioxidants. It may also contribute to the lowering of blood pressure in hypertensive individuals. It contains fiber that may help with regularity and that may also help in lowering blood cholesterol levels.

Collard greens: Contain high levels of antioxidants that are known to contribute to the prevention of several types of cancers. Contain fiber that may contribute to regularity and lower cholesterol levels.

Cranberry: Has antibacterial and antiviral activity. Mostly effective in preventing or alleviating urinary tract infections.

Cucumber: Is a good food for people who are trying to lose weight. It may also help to alleviate certain conditions, including acidosis, constipation, hypertension, mild acne and pimples, and rheumatism.

Eggplant: May help lower bad cholesterol levels, and improve cardiovascular health.

Flax seed: May help to prevent certain cancers. It is useful in relieving constipation. It may lower levels of bad cholesterol, and improve cardiovascular health. It may improve the health and appearance of the skin and reduce the intensity of allergic reactions.

Fig: May help in cancer prevention.

Fish: It is very important to substitute red meat with fish if you are trying to lose weight in a healthy manner. Consume as broad a variety of fish as possible, paying attention to their content of omega-3 fatty acids. Omega-3 fatty acids are the building blocks of fish oil that has been shown to be extremely beneficial to human health. Some common fish such as herring, mackerel, salmon and tuna have very high levels of omega-3 fatty acids. If you absolutely cannot eat fish, you should consider consuming fish oil. The omega-3 fatty acids in fish may help prevent or relieve a variety of cardiovascular, skeletal, respiratory, skin and neuronal conditions. Additionally, some fish contain antioxidants that may be beneficial in cancer prevention.

Grape (red): Contains antioxidant compounds that may contribute to cancer prevention and may improve cardiovascular health. It may lower the levels of bad cholesterol and increase the levels of good cholesterol. The health benefits of consuming red grapes may also be derived from drinking red wine. Of course, you should consult with your doctor prior to engaging in red wine or other types of alcohol.

Grapefruit: Contains antioxidant compounds that may help in cancer prevention and in cardiovascular health.

Kale: Rich in antioxidants that are known to help in cancer prevention.

Mushroom: Some mushrooms such as maitake and shiitake are potent in cancer prevention. They are used for treating cancers in some naturopathic medicines. Also, these mushrooms may lower the levels of bad cholesterol in the blood, help alleviate high blood pressure, and function as a blood thinner. They also have potent anti-viral activities.

Mustard: May help increase the rate of metabolism, resulting in more energy expenditure. It is good for weight loss.

Nuts: Most are rich in antioxidants and are good in preventing cancer and cardiovascular disease. Some nuts such as almonds and walnuts may lower the level of bad cholesterol in the blood. Nuts may contribute to the stabilization of insulin and blood sugar levels, and are therefore a good food for diabetics (type I and type II). An excellent food source for people who are trying to lose weight in a healthy manner.

Oats: May help to lower the levels of bad cholesterol in the blood. It may also help to stabilize blood sugar levels. It is an excellent food for weight loss, and for the regulation of blood cholesterol and blood sugar levels.

Olive oil: This is the oil that you want in your kitchen. It may help improve your cardiovascular health by lowering levels of bad cholesterol, and by blocking the effects of bad cholesterol. It also has antioxidants. As discussed earlier, please use this oil to make infusions of spices for cooking, as condiments, or in salad dressings.

Onion: Rich in antioxidants that have been shown to contribute to the prevention of cancer and cardiovascular disease. The antioxidants in onions are relatively more potent, and onions have been used in some naturopathic medicines as a treatment for some cancers. All types of onions are beneficial, including leeks, scallions, and shallots. Onions may also lower the level of bad cholesterol in blood. Additionally, they may function as a blood thinner and help stabilize blood sugar levels.

Plantain: Plantains (green) are an excellent weight loss food. They should be eaten while they are green.

Pumpkin: Rich in the antioxidant, beta carotene. Just like carrots, pumpkin may contribute to the prevention of cancer and cardiovascular disease. It may also contribute to improved health of the eyes.

Rice: Should be your default source of carbohydrates. May contribute modestly in the prevention of certain cancers. May also lower the level of bad cholesterol in blood.

Seaweed: May help in the prevention of cancer. Individual seaweeds have other health benefits such as the lowering of blood pressure and the level of bad cholesterol in blood. Some may boost the immune system.

Spinach: Spinach is my favorite source of antioxidants. It is loaded with antioxidants that have been shown to contribute in the prevention of cancers and cardiovascular disease. It is also a good source of fiber that may contribute in weight loss and in lowering cholesterol levels. Please eat it raw or only very slightly cooked. Do not strain when cooked.

Strawberry: Has antioxidants that may contribute to the prevention of cancers and cardiovascular disease. Also contains anti-viral activity. Eat strawberries modestly because of their sugar content. They also tend to be contaminated with pesticides.

Tea: Unsweetened tea is a wonderful thing for people who are trying to lose weight in a healthy manner. Replacing soft drinks such as juices and sodas (including diet sodas) with unsweetened tea (black tea, green tea or oolong tea) will contribute visually to weight loss in almost all people. Switching to tea may also improve your cardiovascular health and significantly reduce your chances of developing the metabolic syndrome (type II diabetes and high blood pressure). If you are adversely affected by caffeine, you will enjoy the same health benefits in decaffeinated tea.

Tomato: May help in the prevention of cancers and cardiovascular disease.

Wheat: Whole wheat is rich in fiber. It may help lower the level of bad cholesterol in blood. It may also help in the prevention of certain cancers.

Yams (and sweet potatoes): Contain beta carotene, the antioxidant in carrot and pumpkin. The benefits of this antioxidant include cancer and cardiovascular disease prevention and improved eye health.

Yogurt (unsweetened): Helps boost the immune system. Soothes the stomach and intestines. Good source of calcium – important for bone health.

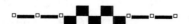

Chapter Three

About Weight Gain, Dieting, and Weight Loss

This chapter is about the fundamentals of weight loss. It is intended to provide a base of knowledge that will allow users of the clinique science weight loss system to make great decisions about weight loss management. Great decisions in weight loss management result in a complete, healthy, and sustainable weight loss. The information in this chapter is particularly important for the following reasons:

1) Weight loss is likely to be more effective in people who understand the source of their obesity. It is important that

you take a minute to identify the possible cause of your obesity prior to starting the clinique science weight loss system – you will get better results. The idea is simple; it is only after understanding the cause of your obesity that you are going to be able to make the little personal lifestyle adjustments that may be necessary to facilitate your weight loss and the maintenance of your new trim look. Take for instance that the cause of your obesity is binge eating – you will only be able to achieve a complete, sustainable and healthy weight loss with the clinique science weight loss system if you make a lifestyle change that addresses the overeating.

2) Knowing how to measure obesity and to recognize the types of obesity will offer you more control in your weight loss. It is important to know your body in terms of where you are most likely to deposit fat, and where fat is shed the fastest while you are on the clinique science weight loss system. The main components of the clinique science weight loss system, medicinal foods and the plateau-proof diet are controllable. It is up to you to determine your desired level of stringency within the recommended guidelines. Of course, as you would expect the rate of weight loss increases with stringency. It is your responsibility to measure your weight profile as accurately as possible, and to make adjustments for accelerating or slowing down the rate of your weight loss as determined by your weight profile.

3) Knowing the basic principles of weight loss dieting is beneficial for completely understanding how the plateau-proof diet works. Since everyone is unique, it is

unreasonable to expect the same diet to have the same efficacy for weight loss in everyone. If everyone knows the fundamentals of weight loss dieting however, everyone will be able to make personal adjustments to increase the efficacy of any weight loss diet. This is also true for the plateau-proof diet.

Obesity

The word obesity originated from the Latin *obesus* (fat). Obesity is an increase in body weight to beyond normal, due to the excess accumulation of fat in the body. How do you know if you are obese, overweight, normal or underweight? The most commonly used standard for measuring obesity today is the body mass index (BMI). Your BMI will give you an approximate body weight profile. More information about BMI is located a few pages ahead along with a BMI chart.

What causes obesity?

Genetics. There is overwhelming evidence that obesity may be passed on from parents to kids. However, just because everyone in your family is obese doesn't necessarily mean that you acquired obesity by heredity. People in the same family may have the same lifestyle or similar behaviors that cause obesity.

Even if the cause of your obesity is genetic you should still be able to enjoy a complete, healthy, and sustainable weight loss with the clinique science weight loss system.

Lifestyle and behaviors. Some of the most common causes of obesity include: what a person eats, how much they eat, eating due to boredom, eating for pleasure (even when not hungry), lack of activity, etc. Honestly evaluate yourself to determine if you may have a problem with one or more of these things. Try to make the necessary adjustments before you start on the clinique science weight loss, and you will have an easier time losing weight.

Psychological factors. Some people react to negative emotions such as sadness, anger, feeling of inadequacy, etc. by overeating. Others react to positive emotions by overeating, and some react to all emotions by overeating. Some people deal with stress by overeating. Some health professionals call this behavior *binge eating disorder*. If you suspect that you may be suffering from this disorder, please see a therapist prior to starting the clinique science weight loss system.

Illnesses. There are certain illnesses that may cause obesity. These illnesses include hypothyroidism, Cushing's syndrome, depression, and other neurological disorders that result in overeating. In most people with obesity induced by illness, the clinique science weight loss system will be effective for attaining and maintaining weight loss.

Drugs. Certain prescription drugs such as steroids and some antidepressants can cause obesity. Relatively very few people become overweight or obese from drug use. If the causative drug is replaceable, that should be done. If the drug is not replaceable, weight loss is still possible (although relatively more difficult) with the clinique science weight loss system.

Are there any health risks associated with obesity?

Obesity is not just about looking big. There are many health risks associated with obesity. A moderately obese person is at least twice as likely as a non-obese person to die prematurely. The risk of premature death increases linearly with weight, or degree and type of obesity. Obesity has been linked to heart disease, stroke, diabetes, high blood pressure, gout, sleep apnea (and other breathing disorders), osteoarthritis, gall bladder disease, gall stones, emotional disorders, colon cancer, rectal cancer, prostate cancer, ovarian cancer, cervical cancer, uterine cancer, breast cancer, cancer of the gall bladder, etc. Apple-shaped obese people are at a higher risk for heart disease, diabetes, and cancer than pear-shaped people of equal weight.

How is obesity measured?

There are many methods available for measuring obesity. It is however sufficient for most people to simply stand on a weight scale. You need to know just one thing when it comes to obesity measurement – the ideal weight range for your height (your normal BMI range). This number is an important number because it forms the core of your weight loss goal(s) on the clinique science weight loss system. It lets you determine when to increase stringency and lose weight and when to decrease stringency and maintain weight.

The body mass index (BMI) is a relatively good method for measuring obesity. This method is fast, simple, reliable, and doesn't require any special equipment. Basically, you match up your weight and height on a BMI chart (see next page) to determine if you are underweight, normal, overweight, or obese. One limitation to the BMI method is that it doesn't take increased muscle mass into account; hence a body builder with a huge muscle mass is likely to have a BMI that indicates that he or she is overweight or obese. If you are not a body builder, the BMI is a reliable method to measure your weight profile.

BMI Chart Weight (lbs) / Height (feet)

Match your height and your weight. If your weight falls in the white (18.5 – 24.9) you are normal, light grey (25 – 29.9) = overweight, and dark grey (above 30) = obese. Below 18.5 = underweight.

NORMAL						OVERWEIGHT					OBESE			
19	20	21	22	23	24	25	26	27	28	29	30	31	32	
														Height
76	80	84	88	92	96	100	104	108	112	116	120	124	128	4' 5"
79	83	87	91	95	100	104	108	112	116	120	124	129	133	4' 6"
82	86	90	95	99	103	108	112	116	120	125	129	133	138	4' 7"
85	89	94	98	103	107	112	116	120	125	129	134	138	143	4' 8"
88	92	97	102	106	111	116	120	125	129	134	139	143	148	4' 9"
91	96	100	105	110	115	120	124	129	134	139	144	148	153	4' 10"
94	99	104	109	114	119	124	129	134	139	144	149	154	158	4' 11"
97	102	108	113	118	123	128	133	138	143	149	154	159	164	5'
101	106	111	116	122	127	132	138	143	148	153	159	164	169	5' 1"
104	109	115	120	126	131	137	142	148	153	159	164	170	175	5' 2"
107	113	119	124	130	135	141	147	152	158	164	169	175	181	5' 3"
111	117	122	128	134	140	146	151	157	163	169	175	181	186	5' 4"
114	120	126	132	138	144	150	156	162	168	174	180	186	192	5' 5"
118	124	130	136	143	149	155	161	167	173	180	186	192	198	5' 6"
121	128	134	140	147	153	160	166	172	179	185	192	198	204	5' 7"
125	132	138	145	151	158	164	171	178	184	191	197	204	210	5' 8"
129	135	142	149	156	163	169	176	183	190	196	203	210	217	5' 9"
132	139	146	153	160	167	174	181	188	195	202	209	216	223	5' 10"
136	143	151	158	165	172	179	186	194	201	208	215	222	229	5' 11"
140	147	155	162	170	177	184	192	199	206	214	221	229	236	6'
144	152	159	167	174	182	190	197	205	212	220	227	235	243	6' 1"
148	156	164	171	179	187	195	203	210	218	226	234	241	249	6' 2"
152	160	168	176	184	192	200	208	216	224	232	240	248	256	6' 3"
156	164	173	181	189	197	205	214	222	230	238	246	255	263	6' 4"
160	169	177	186	194	202	211	219	228	236	245	253	261	270	6' 5"
164	173	182	190	199	208	216	225	234	242	251	260	268	277	6' 6"
169	178	186	195	204	213	222	231	240	249	257	266	275	284	6' 7"
173	182	191	200	209	218	228	237	246	255	264	273	282	291	6' 8"
177	187	196	205	215	224	233	243	252	261	271	280	289	299	6' 9"
182	191	201	210	220	230	239	249	258	268	277	287	297	306	6' 10"
186	196	206	216	225	235	245	255	265	274	284	294	304	314	6' 11"
191	201	211	221	231	241	251	261	271	281	291	301	311	321	7'
195	206	216	226	236	247	257	267	277	288	298	308	319	329	7' 1"
200	210	221	231	242	252	263	274	284	295	305	316	326	337	7' 2"

205	215	226	237	248	258	269	280	291	301	312	323	334	345	7' 3"
209	220	231	242	253	264	275	286	297	308	319	330	341	353	7' 4"
214	225	237	248	259	270	282	293	304	315	327	338	349	361	7' 5"
219	230	242	253	265	277	288	300	311	323	334	346	357	369	7' 6"

BMI Chart Weight (Kg) / Height (meters)

Match your height and your weight. If your weight falls in the white (18.5 – 24.9) you are normal, light grey (25 – 29.9) = overweight, and dark grey (above 30) = obese. Below 18.5 = underweight.

	NORMAL					OVERWEIGHT					OBESE			
19	20	21	22	23	24	25	26	27	28	29	30	31	32	
														Height
19	20	21	22	23	24	25	26	27	28	29	30	31	32	1.0
23	24	25	27	28	29	30	31	33	34	35	36	38	39	1.1
27	29	30	32	33	35	36	37	39	40	42	43	45	46	1.2
32	34	35	37	39	41	42	44	46	47	49	51	52	54	1.3
37	39	41	43	45	47	49	51	53	55	57	59	61	63	1.4
43	45	47	50	52	54	56	59	61	63	65	68	70	72	1.5
49	51	54	56	59	61	64	67	69	72	74	77	79	82	1.6
55	58	61	64	66	69	72	75	78	81	84	87	90	92	1.7
62	65	68	71	75	78	81	84	87	91	94	97	100	104	1.8
69	72	76	79	83	87	90	94	97	101	105	108	112	116	1.9
76	80	84	88	92	96	100	104	108	112	116	120	124	128	2.0
84	88	93	97	101	106	110	115	119	123	128	132	137	141	2.1
92	97	102	106	111	116	121	126	131	136	140	145	150	155	2.2
101	106	111	116	122	127	132	138	143	148	153	159	164	169	2.3
109	115	121	127	132	138	144	150	156	161	167	173	179	184	2.4
119	125	131	138	144	150	156	163	169	175	181	188	194	200	2.5
128	135	142	149	155	162	169	176	183	189	196	203	210	216	2.6
139	146	153	160	168	175	182	190	197	204	211	219	226	233	2.7
149	157	165	172	180	188	196	204	212	220	227	235	243	251	2.8
160	168	177	185	193	202	210	219	227	235	244	252	261	269	2.9
171	180	189	198	207	216	225	234	243	252	261	270	279	288	3.0

The most accurate method for measuring obesity involves weighing a person under water. This method is complicated and requires the use of sophisticated equipment. Other less accurate methods include measuring skin fold thickness in many areas of the body, and bioelectric impedance analysis – a technique in which small electrical currents are sent through the body. For most people however, the BMI is a reasonably reliable measuring technique.

The waist-to-hip ratio

The waist-to-hip ratio is used to determine if a person is apple-shaped or pear-shaped. Most disease risk factors are greater in apple-shaped obesity than in pear-shaped obesity. To get the waist-to-hip ratio, measure the waist at the narrowest point (x) and measure the hips at the widest point (y). Divide (x) by (y) [x/y] – this is your waist-to-hip ratio. If you are a woman with a ratio greater than 0.8 you are apple-shaped, and less than 0.8 you are pear-shaped. If you are a man with a ratio greater than 1.0 you are apple-shaped, and less than 1.0 you are pear-shaped. Again, if you are apple-shaped, you are at a greater risk for cardiovascular disease and other diseases. You would benefit the most from rapid weight loss, so you may want to follow the clinique science weight loss system stringently.

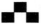

The main types of weight loss diets, the rationales behind them and how well they work

1) *Hypocaloric diets.* These are weight loss diets that restrict the amount of calories allowed per day (low calorie diets). The rationale behind these diets is to consume less energy than the amount of energy required by the body. In other words, you will lose weight if you take in less energy than you spend. In a rather simplistic way, it appears logical that the balance of the energy is going to come from energy stores (fat) in the body. This is also the rationale of people who try to attain complete weight loss by exercising vigorously. These diets typically affect an initial weight loss in most people. The weight loss eventually hits a plateau, after which people tend to relapse into weight gain[132,133]. Although the hypocaloric diet rationale is logical, it doesn't consider that the human body is not the same as a combustion engine; hence the laws of thermodynamics break down rapidly when applied to the human body. In other words, there are many other factors to consider in the functioning of the human body beyond a difference in energy expended and energy consumed. It is for this reason that hypocaloric diets affect a weight loss that plateaus relatively rapidly.

2) *The low-carb and very low-carb diets.* These are low calorie diets in which the energy restriction is due to a decrease in the amount of carbohydrates in the diets. Some popular low-carb diets substitute the carbs for fat. There is no consensus as to what amount of carbs distinguishes the low-carb diets from the very low-carb diets, so for the

purposes of this book, I will use 'low-carb' to refer to both. These diets are effective for short-term weight loss, but the weight loss reaches a plateau relatively quicker than with other diets[134-144]. Some of these diets allow for unrestricted amounts of saturated fats, and are potentially dangerous for cardiovascular health. These diets probably fail to affect a complete weight loss or to maintain lost weight because they are one dimensional – they simply restrict the amount of one macronutrient – carbohydrate. There are too many factors involved in metabolism, weight gain and weight loss, suggesting that a one dimensional diet is unlikely to provide a long term solution to weight loss.

3) *Low-fat diets.* The low-fat diets are also hypocaloric diets in which the energy restriction is from decreasing the amount of fat. Low-fat diets affect weight loss at a slower rate than the low-carb diets; however, the weight loss reaches a plateau slower than with the low-carb diets[136,138,145-154].

4) *Ketogenic diets.* The ketogenic diets are very low calorie diets that cause an increase in the level of ketones in the blood (ketosis)[153-156]. The ketones come from the metabolism of fat, since these diets are typically high in fat and low in carbs. The ketones also come from the fat that is stored in the body. Ketosis makes the blood more acidic (reduce the pH of blood). Ketosis is essentially a state of blood toxicity (poisoning). It is believed that sustained ketosis may cause metabolic disorders as well as problems with the liver and kidneys. Ketosis typically occurs with very low-carb diets. Some proponents of low-carb diets believe that the increase in blood ketones causes suppression of

appetite; however, results from medical studies do not agree with that claim[134].

5) *High-fiber diets*. These diets reduce the amount of glucose absorbed into the blood stream by increasing the amount of indigestible carbs (fiber). Since humans are incapable of digesting fiber, the fiber contributes to the bulk of the diet but not to its energy value. High-fiber diets can contribute to a limited extent in the treatment of obesity[157-170]. Diets rich in fiber have been shown to be beneficial for the health, including the facilitation of bowel movements and a reduction in the risk of certain cancers[171-188]. Some types of fiber can help to lower the levels of bad cholesterol in the blood. Although they are not efficient for weight loss by themselves high-fiber diets are healthy and they should be a part of all weight loss diets. The plateau-proof diet uses a fiber index to incorporate foods that are rich in fiber.

6) *The protein-sparing diets.* Also called the protein-sparing modified fast, these diets typically allow only meats, fish and vegetables[189-205]. These are very low-carb hypocaloric diets that require close medical monitoring as they can cause severe ketosis and cardiac arrhythmia (a type of heart failure)[206]. Initial weight loss is typically rapid, but these diets are obviously unsustainable.

7) Low glycemic load diets. Low glycemic load diets are similar to high-fiber diets[207]. The low glycemic load diets also select carbohydrates with low energy densities. What distinguishes the low glycemic load diets from the high-fiber diets is that the low glycemic load diets emphasize the rate of absorption of glucose into the bloodstream. In other

words, these diets favor carbohydrates that are more slowly digested and absorbed as glucose into the bloodstream. In terms of weight loss, the low glycemic load diets seem to have no advantage over the high-fiber diets. Low glycemic load diets however may have an advantage over regular high-carbohydrate diets in obese patients with type II diabetes. Glucose metabolism is impaired in type II diabetes, making the blood glucose levels higher than normal. Since the low glycemic load diets release glucose into the bloodstream at a slower pace, they may help control the level of glucose in the blood.

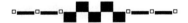

The showdown – Low-carb diets versus low-fat diets

Low-carb diets are popular nowadays, with many Fad dieters using different variations of it. Low-carb diets have actually been around since the 1800s, and have been used therapeutically for the management of obesity. William Banting, for example, described his low-carb diet in the 1860s[208]. Banting, who was 66 years old at the time, claimed to have benefited from appetite suppression from the diet, and a resultant weight loss of 46 pounds (initial weight was 202 lbs) in a one year period. He praised the diet for having an immediate effect; noticeable within a week.

We are a long way from Banting's days; however, the efficacy (effectiveness) and safety of low-carb diets are still a matter of debate and controversy. Proponents of the low-carb diets claim that these diets are relatively more effective for weight loss compared to low-fat diets. Others claim that these diets can be used to cure obesity (as in get thin and stay thin). Opponents of the low-carb diets dispute the long-term efficacy and safety of these diets. They claim that these diets are likely to cause abnormalities in metabolism, which will lead to liver and kidney disease.

This section looks at the results several clinical studies on the efficacy and safety of low-carb and low-fat diets. For simplicity some of the clinical studies are summarized in tables, and each table is followed by a brief discussion of the study. They are included here to give you an indication of which of the two macronutrients (carbohydrate or fat) is a better target for weight loss.

Table 1. Low-carb diet.

Location / year of study	Virginia Polytechnic Institute, Blacksburg, VA USA. 2005
Diet type	*Very low-carb (20 g per day for 2 weeks followed by an increase of 5 g per week for 10 weeks).*
Average weight loss	*8.3% of initial body weight – 7 Kg (15.4 lbs)*
Duration of study	*12 weeks*
Number of participants	*13*
Special considerations	*Study monitored blood and urine ketone levels. Ketone levels increased in week 1, then dropped progressively.*

This trial[134] studied the effects of a very low-carbohydrate diet on 13 premenopausal women between the ages of 32 and 45. The study was done in an out-patient setting. The average initial weight of the participants was 84.8 Kg (186.9 lbs). Average weight loss at 12 weeks was 7 Kg (15.4 lbs). Prior to the start of the low-carb diet, the average energy from food for these women was 2,025 Kcal per day (49% carbs, 15% protein, 36% fats). Energy consumption at week 1 was 1,290 cal per day (10% carbs, 32% proteins, 57% fats), and at week 12 was 1,535 cal per day (15% carbs, 24% proteins, 61% fats).

The results of this study show a short-term decrease in body weight resulting from a low-carb diet. The duration of the study was too short to determine if further weight loss could be attained. Equally, the duration of the study was not long enough to determine if the weight loss could be maintained, or if there was relapse into weight gain. The study did not address any safety parameters, but also did not report any immediate health complications from the participants.

Table 2. Low-carb diet.

Location / year of study	University of Witwatersrand, Johannesburg, South Africa. 2000.
Diet type	Low-carb – 1600 Kcal (40% carbs, 30% proteins, 30% fats). Refined carbs were replaced with complex carbs. Saturated fats were replaced with unsaturated fats.
Average weight loss	7.7 Kg (17 lbs)
Duration of study	16 weeks
Number of participants	13
Special considerations	All participants were gout patients.

This trial[141] studied the effects of a low-carbohydrate diet on 13 men between the ages of 38 and 62. The average weight of the participants at the beginning of the study was 91.1Kg (200.8 lbs), and average weight at 16 weeks was 83.4 Kg (183.7 lbs). Average weight loss at 16 weeks was 7.7 Kg (17 lbs). Participants decreased their dietary carbs, replacing them with proteins. Daily protein consumption was around 120 g. Dairy intake was limited as a source of protein, while poultry and fish were added in the diet to increase protein.

In addition to the weight loss, this low-carbohydrate diet also decreased fat and cholesterol levels in the blood. Blood levels of triglycerides (fat) dropped from 4.7 mmol/l to 1.9 mmol/l. Blood levels of LDL cholesterol (bad cholesterol) dropped from 3.5 mmol/l to 2.7 mmol/l in 16 weeks.

The results of this study suggest that short-term weight loss can be attained with a diet that is low in carbs. It goes further to show that a diet low in carbs and saturated fat, and high in protein may decrease risk factors (triglycerides and LDL-C) for heart disease. The duration of the study is however too short to draw any inferences for the long-term. Also, the sample size (number of participants in the study) is too small for the study to stand on its own.

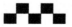

Table 3. Low-carb vs low-fat diet.

Location / year of study	*Multicenter – headed in University of Pennsylvania School of Med. USA. 2003*
Diet type	*Very low-carb – 20 g / day in the first 2 weeks and gradual increase. No restriction in fats and proteins.*
Average weight loss	*9.6 Kg (21.2 lbs) after 6 months* *7.2 Kg (15.9 lbs) after 12 months*
Duration of study	*12 months*
Number of participants	*63 (20 males & 43 females)*
Special considerations	*The study compared the efficacy of a low-carb diet to that of the conventional low-fat diet.*

This study[135] involved two groups of participants – one on a very low-carb diet with no restrictions in fats and proteins, and the other on a conventional low-fat, hypocaloric (low calorie) diet. In the low-carb group, carb intake was limited to 20 g per day in the first 2 weeks of the study, and then slowly increased. The other group had a high-carb, low-fat diet with energy restrictions – 1200-1500 Kcal and 1500-1800 Kcal per day respectively for men and women. The diet was composed of about 60% carbs, 25% fats and 15% proteins. Age and obesity levels were similar in both groups.

The low-carb group lost weight faster than the conventional low-fat diet group – 21.2 lbs compared to 11.5 lbs at six months into the study. This difference was smaller at 12 months into the study, with the low-carb group climbing to 15.9 lbs and the conventional diet group remaining almost unchanged at 9.7 lbs.

There was a significant decrease in the blood triglyceride (fat) levels in the low-carb group, which was sustained to the 12 month point. There wasn't a similar decrease in blood triglyceride levels in the low-fat diet group. The low-fat diet group however had a decrease in LDL-C (bad cholesterol) levels, which was not witnessed in the low-carb group. The lowering of both triglycerides and LDL-C in the low-carb group from *table 2*, was then likely due to the substitution of saturated fats with unsaturated fats and protein.

The dropout rate was high in this study, with only 59% of participants completing the study. The results of this study suggest that a low-carb diet may be more effective than a low-fat diet for short-term weight loss. We see however that the low-carb diet reached a weight loss plateau after six months. After the plateau, there was relapse into weight gain (21.2 lbs lost after 6 months and 15.9 lbs lost after 12 months). The low-fat diet also hit a plateau by 12 months (11.5 lbs lost after 6 months and 9.7 lbs after 12 months).

Obesity is a chronic condition; therefore, dieting can only be an effective therapy if the diet is not limited by the weight loss plateau.

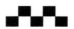

Table 4. Low-carb vs low-fat diet.

Location / year of study	University of Illinois at Urbana-Champaign. USA. 2003
Diet type	Low-carb low-fat – 1700 Kcal/day (30% proteins, 41% carbs, 29% fats)
Average weight loss	7.5 Kg (16.5 lbs)
Duration of study	10 weeks
Number of participants	24
Special considerations	This study compared a low-fat, low-carb diet to a low-fat, high-carb diet. 12 participants in each group.

The participants in this study[142] were 24 females ages 45 to 65. The study compared the effects of a low-carb diet to those of a low-fat, high-carb diet over a 10 week period. The low-carb diet consisted of 30% proteins, 41% carbs, and 29% fats, while the higher carb diet consisted of 16% proteins, 58% carbs, and 26% fat. Average weight loss in the low-carb group was 7.5 Kg (16. 5 lbs), compared to 6.96 Kg (15.3 lbs) in the higher carb group. The ratio of fat to lean tissue (muscle) loss was higher in the low-carb group.

The results of this study suggest that low-carb diets cause a more rapid short-term weight loss than low-fat diets. These results cannot be extrapolated to the long-term, since the trial time was too short. It however compliments other studies, which have shown that low-carb diets are more effective than low-fat diets for short-term weight loss.

Table 5. Low-carb diet.

Location / year of study	Multicenter – Glasgow and Aberdeen, UK. 1996
Diet type	Low-carb – 1200 Kcal (35% of energy from carbs).
Average weight loss	5.6 Kg (12.3 lbs) at 3 months 6.8 Kg (14.9 lbs) at 6 months
Duration of study	6 months
Number of participants	110
Special considerations	Study compared low-carb and high-carb diet for weight loss and cardiovascular risk factors.

This study[143] involved 110 women ages 18 to 68. The women were divided into 2 groups; one group was placed on a low-carb diet and the other on a high-carb diet. Both diets provided the same amount of calories (1200 Kcal per day). In the low-carb diet, carbs contributed 35% of the calories, while in the high-carb diet; carbs contributed 58% of the calories. At 3 months, the high-carb group lost an average of 4.3 Kg (9.5 lbs) and the low-carb group lost an average of 5.6 Kg (12.3 lbs). In the high-carb group, total cholesterol level in the blood was lowered as were levels of LDL-C (bad cholesterol). In the low-carb group, total triglycerides (fat) were lowered, but there was no improvement in blood cholesterol levels.

At 6 months, the high-carb group lost an average of 5.6 Kg (12.3 lbs), and the low-carb group lost an average of 6.8 Kg (14.9 lbs). Blood cholesterol levels remained lower in the high-carb group, and blood triglyceride levels were lowered too. In the low-carb group, blood triglyceride levels stayed lower, however there was no improvement in total blood cholesterol levels, and other risk factors for cardiovascular disease.

The results from this study indicate that short-term weight loss can be attained using either a high-carb or low-carb diet. These results also suggest that there is another factor (other than the lowering of carbs) that affects weight loss. We are going to see later that this factor is protein. Weight loss with the low-carb diet was more rapid than weight loss with the high-carb diet, which is consistent with the results of the previously discussed studies. The risk factors for cardiovascular disease were improved on the high-carb diet, but not on the low-carb diet. This indicates that low-carb diets with unrestricted fat intake may pose a risk to cardiovascular health.

Table 6. Low-carb vs low-fat diet.

Location / year of study	University of Guelph, Ontario, Canada. 2004
Diet type	Very low-carb – very low energy (766.8 Kcal/day) - 15.4% of energy intake from carbs.
Average weight loss	7.0 Kg (15.4 lbs)
Duration of study	10 weeks
Number of participants	31
Special considerations	This study compared a very low-carb and low-fat diet for weight loss and cardiovascular disease risk factors.

This study[136] involved 31 men and women 24 to 61 years old. The 10 week study compared the effect of a very low-carb and a low-fat diet on weight loss and blood levels of cardiovascular disease risk factors. Total energy from food was extremely low in both diets – 766.8 Kcal per day for the very low-carb diet, and 609.6 Kcal per day for the low-fat diet. At 10 weeks, the very low-carb group lost an average of 7.0 Kg (15.4 lbs), and the low-fat group lost an average of 6.8 Kg (14.9 lbs). This study, like the others, supports the observation that low-carb diets provide a faster rate of weight loss than low-fat diets. It is important to note that the previous studies compared diets that provided the same daily amounts of calories (isocaloric diets). In this study, the low-fat diet had fewer calories than the low-carb diet; however, weight loss was greater in the low-carb group than in the low-fat group. This shows that weight loss is not just a matter of calories, and the management of weight loss should not be limited to caloric restriction.

The other results of this study showed an improvement in cardiovascular risk factors in the low-fat group, but not in the low-carb group. Total cholesterol and LDL-C (bad cholesterol) were lowered in the low-fat group at 10 weeks. This is consistent with the findings in the previous studies, supporting the observation that low-fat diets are superior to low-carb diets (with unrestricted fat) in lowering the risk factors of cardiovascular disease.

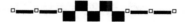

Table 7. Low-carb vs low-fat diet.

Location / year of study	Sakura Hospital, School of Medicine, Japan. 2003
Diet type	Low-carb (1000 Kcal / day total energy with 25% proteins, 40% carbs, and 35% fats).
Average weight loss	9.0 Kg (19.8 lbs)
Duration of study	4 weeks
Number of participants	22
Special considerations	This study compared a low-carb diet and a low-fat diet for weight loss and visceral (gut) fat in obese diabetes patients.

The participants in this study[144] were 22 obese diabetes patients. They were divided into 2 groups, and placed on either a low-carb diet or a low-fat diet. Both diets provided an equal amount (1000 Kcal) of daily energy (isocaloric). The low-carb diet consisted of 25% protein, 40% carbs and 35% fats. The low-fat diet consisted of 25% protein, 65% carbs, and 10% fats. At 4 weeks, the low-carb group lost an average of 9.0 Kg (19.8 lbs) and the low-fat group lost an average of 7.0 Kg (15.4 lbs). The quantity of visceral (gut) fat was also measured. The low-carb group lost 4 times more visceral fat than the low-fat group.

The results of this study are consistent with those of previous studies which show that low-carb diets are superior to low-fat diets for attaining short-term weight loss. Like some of the other studies we have discussed, the duration of this study (4 weeks) was too short to extrapolate the long-term effects.

This study however suggests an important characteristic of low-carb–induced weight loss. It shows that there may be more targeting and reduction of visceral fat with low-carb diets than with low-fat diets. Other studies have supported this finding. The significance of this is that a more rapid reduction of visceral fat will more quickly lower the risk of some obesity-related diseases. Previous studies showed that certain cardiovascular risk factors are reduced with low-fat diets, but not with low-carb diets. This and other studies suggest that low-carb diets may have their own selective ability in lowering disease risk by rapidly decreasing visceral fat. Since the weight loss from low-carb diets plateaus rapidly, this protection is only for the short term.

Table 8. Low-carb vs low-fat diet.

Location / year of study	Philadelphia VA Medical Center, USA. 2003
Diet type	Low-carb with total carbs limited to under 30 g per day.
Average weight loss	5.8 Kg (12.8 lbs)
Duration of study	6 months
Number of participants	132
Special considerations	This study compared the effects of a low-carb diet and a low-fat diet on weight loss.

This study[138] compared the weight loss efficiency of a low-carb versus a low-fat diet. There were 132 participants in this study. A significant number of the participants had either diabetes or the metabolic syndrome. The minimum age of the participants was 18. The low-carb group had no restrictions on fat intake, but was instructed to limit carbs to 30 g per day or less. This group was also advised to consume fruits and vegetables with high-fiber content. The low-fat group had 30% or less of total daily calories from fat. At 6 months, the low-carb group lost an average of 5.8 Kg (12.8 lbs), and the low-fat group lost an average of 1.9 Kg (4.1 lbs).

The results of this study support those of the previous studies, showing that low-carb diets are more efficient than low-fat diets for short-term weight loss.

Table 9. Low-carb vs low-fat diet.

Location / year of study	Multicenter – U. of Pennsylvania Health System, USA. 2004
Diet type	Low-carb – not more than 30 g per of carbs. Diet consisted of 25% proteins, 32% carbs, and 43% fats.
Average weight loss	8.5 Kg (18.7 lbs)
Duration of study	6 months
Number of participants	78
Special considerations	This study compared the weight loss efficiency of a low-carb diet and a low-fat diet.

78 participants completed this 6 month study[139]. The study compared the weight loss efficiency of a low-carb diet and a low-fat diet. 35 participants completed the low-fat program, and 43

participants completed the low-carb program. Participants in the low-carb group consumed no more than 30 g of carbs per day. The diet in the low-carb group consisted of 25% proteins, 32% carbs, and 43% fats. Participants in the low-fat group had around 30% or less of total daily calories from fats. Their diet consisted of 16% protein, 32% carbs and 43% fats.

At 6 months, the low-carb group lost an average of 8.5 Kg (18.7 lbs), and the low-fat group lost an average of 3.5 Kg (7.7 lbs). The study also measured levels of C-reactive protein (an indicator of inflammation) in the body. There was no significant difference between the 2 groups for levels of C-reactive protein. There was however a difference among the high risk (for inflammation) participants. Among the high risk participants, the low-carb diet showed a greater decrease in the levels of C-reactive protein than the low-fat diet. This indicates that a low-carb diet may be more efficient in reducing the risk of inflammation in high risk obese patients.

The results of this study support those of previous studies in showing that low-carb diets are more efficient than low-fat diets for short-term weight loss. The fact that low-carb diets may reduce inflammation, shows another benefit of low-carb diets that is lacking in conventional low-fat diets. Of course, we have to be mindful of the fact that low-carb diets with unrestricted fat intake pose a serious risk to cardiovascular health. We also have to be mindful of the fact that weight loss affected by low-carb diets is short-term, and it is equally likely that the reduction of inflammation risks may also be short-term – coinciding with the duration of weight loss.

Table 10. Low-carb vs low-fat diet.

Location / year of study	Philadelphia VA Medical Center, USA. 2004
Diet type	Low-carb with total carbs limited to under 30 g per day.
Average weight loss	5.1 Kg (11.2 lbs)
Duration of study	12 months
Number of participants	132
Special considerations	This study compared the effects of a low-carb diet and a low-fat diet on weight loss.

This study[140] was a follow-up study from the study in *Table 8.* The study compared the efficacy of a low-carb diet versus a conventional low-fat diet for weight loss. The initial study was reported at 6 months from the start of the diet program. This study shows weight loss figures at 12 months. At 12 months, the low-carb group lost an average of 5.1 Kg (11.2 lbs), compared to 5.8 Kg (12.8 lbs) at 6 months. The low-fat group lost an average of 3.1 Kg (6.8 lbs) at 12 months, compared to 1.9 Kg (4.1 lbs) at 6 months. The results of this study show that although the low-carb diets have a rapid effect on weight loss, they are ineffective in causing additional weight loss in the longer term (plateau). The low-fat diets on the other hand, do not show a rapid effect on weight loss; however, their weight loss effect is sustained over a longer period of time. It takes longer for weight loss to plateau with low-fat diets compared to low-carb diets. The results of these weight loss diets are representative of the trends in the population at large. The major frustration in weight loss dieting reported by most people is incomplete weight loss due to the weight loss plateau, and the inability to maintain lost weight.

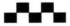

And the winner is...

The clear winner is low-carb diets, that is, if you are comparing short term weight loss. If on the other hand, you are comparing first to plateau, the winner is low-fat diets. If you are comparing improvement in cardiovascular parameters such as the lowering of triglycerides and LDC cholesterol; both low-carb and low-fat diets need help. The help comes in the form of protein – more on that later.

In comparing low-carb and low-fat diets, low-carb diets affected a bigger weight loss even when the low-fat diets had significantly fewer calories. This finding indicates that the amount of calories consumed in a diet is not as important for weight loss as is the macronutrient composition of the diet. In other words, the relative amount of carbohydrates, fats, and proteins in a diet is more important for weight loss than counting calories. To borrow from George Orwell – It appears that all calories are equal but some are more equal than others. If the human body was a combustion engine then the source of the calories wouldn't matter. We are a little more complex than engines though and the source of the calories clearly matters. Firstly, recall from the metabolism charts that each macronutrient has a distinct metabolic pathway with different rates of burn versus store. Also, the metabolism of carbohydrates and fats is compromised during obesity further complicating the efficiency of weight loss from a strictly caloric perspective.

The clinical studies also show that weight loss reaches a plateau significantly faster with the low-carb diets than with the low-fat diets. This suggests that the body adapts to the low-carb diets faster than it adapts to the low-fat diets. This also indicates that the adaptation of the body to resist further weight loss is not dependent on the amount of calories in the diet. Since the low-fat diets had more calories, one would expect them to trigger the weight loss plateau faster than the low-carb diets if the amount of calories consumed was a significant factor. These findings bring to light an important limitation of the hypocaloric diets. **_Due to this limitation, the counting of calories is not a part of the plateau-proof diet (presented in the next chapter)._**

—

Are low-carb diets safe?

Results from several clinical trials that compared low-carb diets to low-fat diets raise a serious concern about the safety of low-carb diets. In the low-carb diet studies where fat was unrestricted, the level of LDL-C (bad cholesterol) in the blood was elevated, while blood levels of HDL-C (good cholesterol) was decreased or unchanged. The increase in the blood levels of bad cholesterol in low-carb diets presents a risk for cardiovascular disease. Low-carb diets that place no restriction on fats (particularly saturated fats and trans fats) are therefore dangerous, presenting an increased risk of cardiovascular disease and other diseases. The low-carb diets however showed some beneficial effects on health, in addition to weight loss. Some studies showed that visceral (gut) fat is preferentially and more rapidly reduced with low-carb diets than with the conventional low-fat diets. Gut fat presents a greater risk of cardiovascular disease than fat located elsewhere in the body. Low-carb diets have also been shown to reduce the chances of inflammation in obese people who are most at risk of it. In terms of safety therefore, low-carb diets appear to be safe when saturated fats and trans fats are restricted.

The role of protein

When it comes to dieting for weight loss, protein is the key. There is an abundance of research data in favor of increasing the amount of protein consumed in weight loss diets[146,147,150,153,209-225]. The first thing to consider is that once you gain weight, your body does not metabolize carbohydrates and fats as well as it did before you gained weight, but it still metabolizes protein normally. The cells that make up your body become inefficient in picking up carbs (glucose) and fats from blood, and they also become inefficient in burning glucose and fat for energy. There is rather an increased tendency to convert glucose into fat, which is stored in fat cells along with excess dietary fat. An overweight body is therefore inclined to gain more weight. This type of situation is referred to as a positive feedback mechanism, and could easily lead to morbid obesity. Not to worry, the right type and right amount of proteins in the diet can break this positive feedback mechanism and place you on track for a complete and sustainable weight loss. Here are some of the things the right type of proteins can do:

- The induction of thermogenesis (an energy consuming process during which the body produces heat). The increase in thermogenesis causes an increase in the expenditure of energy that would otherwise be stored as fat. Studies have shown that the rate of consumption of dietary energy is significantly higher when the diet is high in protein[214,218,223,224,226-230]. This phenomenon is called diet-induced thermogenesis (DIT). It is mainly due to proteins, as DIT from the other macronutrients is insignificant for weight loss. This energy is used to generate heat. It is a desirable thing to lose excess energy as heat, rather than store it as fat.

- More satiety (fullness) with a high-protein diet than with a high-fat diet. People tend to get full faster on a high-protein diet than on a high-fat diet[223,224]. This advantage of a high-protein diet cannot be overemphasized. A lot of obesity is caused by, or aggravated by overeating. A protein-rich diet may help with portion control by making you feel full with relatively smaller portions.

- A more favorable cardiovascular profile, in terms of lowering the risk factors of heart disease[147,150,217]. Whereas diets high in fat, particularly saturated fats, have been shown to increase the risk for heart disease, high-protein diets have been shown to have a favorable effect on the risk of heart disease and other diseases.

- Proteins may increase the rate of burning stored fat. Studies have shown that higher levels of protein in the diet increase the rate of breakdown of fat that is stored in fat cells[231,232].

- A high-protein diet is particularly effective in decreasing gut fat. This is another way in which a high-protein diet will contribute to a favorable cardiovascular profile. Additionally, it provides the esthetic value of a good waist to hip ratio.

- Long-term safety. High-protein diets are safe for long-term use[146,147,212]. This is true when the right type of proteins are consumed in the diet, and balanced with the right type of carbohydrates and fats.

- Increased protein in the diet may trigger the secretion of growth hormone during weight loss[233-236]. Growth hormone helps the adult body to stay lean, and its secretion is suppressed in obesity[237]. Growth hormone secretion may be regained with weight loss[233,238]. If growth hormone secretion is regained after weight loss, it is easier to maintain the new lean figure. If weight loss is not accompanied by the secretion of growth hormone, there is likely to be a relapse into weight gain. Not all weight loss diets trigger growth hormone secretion with weight loss[239]. The evidence suggests that high-protein diets trigger the secretion of growth hormone during weight loss.

What type of proteins should you eat then? What type of carbohydrates and fats should you balance the proteins with? In trying to answer this question in a manner that will be useful to the greatest number of people in terms of consistency in weight loss, there must be a means of standardizing the carbohydrates and fats to the proteins. By standardizing, I mean numbers. You may have standardized your diet in the past by counting calories; here the standardization will consider macronutrient composition. Macronutrient composition is considered rather than calories because it is more significant for weight loss than counting calories. How do we standardize?

The best solution is to take what we know about the macronutrients and weight loss and create a mathematical formula that holds everything together. With such a formula, we can eliminate or greatly minimize the inconsistencies in weight loss and make weight loss more predictable, more robust and more sustainable. After coming up with that formula, every food on the planet can be plugged into the formula and assigned a number that will let you know whether or not you can eat that food. This may sound complicated but don't worry because I have already plugged in the foods to the formula, assigned numbers to the foods, and arranged them in tables. I called this the plateau-proof diet because it should affect a complete weight loss in most people when used correctly.

The Plateau-proof Diet

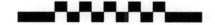

The science behind the plateau-proof diet

Based on the fact that protein is the only macronutrient that has a relatively normal metabolism during obesity and that protein can actively contribute to weight loss (see previous chapter), the plateau proof diet uses protein as a standard to classify carbohydrates and fats. Two mathematical formulas (CP formula and FP formula) are used for this standardization. The formulas assign numbers to foods – the lower the number the better a food is for weight loss. The mathematical formulas and an explanation of how they were derived are discussed in the next section. Assigning numbers to foods is essential for weight loss because it gives you control by letting you know what foods to eat to lose weight fast and what foods to eat to lose weight slowly. Remember that neither the amount of calories nor the amount of food eaten is as important for weight loss as the type of food eaten. By type of food eaten, I mean the macronutrient composition of the food, and the health factors as shown in the CP and FP formulas. For your convenience the foods are arranged in 3 tables (a green, a yellow, and a red table) along with their numbers. The green table has the best foods for weight loss, and the red table contains foods that should be avoided. The yellow table contains foods that are between the green and the red.

The plateau-proof diet is composed of a high-protein low-carb component (CP rotation) that alternates with a high-protein low-fat component (FP rotation). The reason for this rotation is to avoid or minimize the weight loss plateau. It is this component of the diet that inspired its name. Weight loss in the CP rotation of the diet is relatively rapid, but it also will reach a plateau relatively rapidly. To avoid the plateau, you will switch to the FP rotation while you are still at the peak of weight loss in the CP rotation (4 weeks). Your weight loss is going to be slower in the FP rotation, but it shouldn't plateau. Once your body adapts to the FP rotation (2 weeks), you will switch to the CP rotation and restart the process. You will continue to alternate between the CP and FP rotations until you achieve complete weight loss. When you have achieved complete weight loss, you may reduce the stringency of the diet and the rotations as is required to maintain your lean body.

The plateau-proof diet formulas (The CP formula and the FP formula)

The first of the two formulas is called the CP (carb/protein) formula and the second is called the FP (fat/protein) formula.

The CP and FP formulas in the most basic sense ensure that no carbs or fats enter the body unaccompanied by the right protein. I already discussed why we need protein for a complete and sustainable weight loss in the previous chapter, but I am going to state the reasons again:

1) Protein is the only macronutrient that has normal metabolism in obesity. The metabolism of both fat and carbohydrate is compromised and deficient.

2) Protein triggers thermogenesis shortly after it is eaten. The body burns energy as heat during the process of thermogenesis. In the absence of thermogenesis, this energy would be stored as fat in the body. Since neither carbs nor fat induce thermogenesis, it is not such a bright idea swallowing them down without the right amount of protein.

3) Protein may trigger the secretion of growth hormone during weight loss. Growth hormone secretion is essential to maintain a lean body. In obesity, the secretion of growth hormone is compromised, and the blood level of growth hormone drops. Weight loss by itself may not trigger the release of growth hormone; however, weight loss on a high-protein diet may trigger release of growth hormone. It is easier to lose weight and to maintain a new lean body when growth hormone is present in the blood.

4) Proteins may increase the rate of burning of stored fat. Studies have shown that with a high protein diet, the protein may increase the rate of breakdown of fat that is stored in fat cells, thereby contributing to weight loss.

5) A high-protein weight loss diet is particularly effective in decreasing gut (visceral) fat. This is another way in which a high-protein diet will contribute to a favorable cardiovascular profile. Additionally, it provides the esthetic value of a good waist to hip ratio.

6) Diets rich in protein affect satiety (feeling of fullness) faster, hence minimizing the risk of over eating.

7) High-protein diets are safe for long-term use when balanced with the right type and right amounts of carbohydrates and fats.

For these reasons, protein is at the core of the plateau-proof diet, with the CP and FP formulas tagging dietary carbohydrates and fats to protein.

■

Derivation of the CP formula

The first step in the derivation of the CP formula considers the number of calories provided by 1 gram of protein and 1 gram of carbs. It starts by multiplying the number of calories to number of grams.

Therefore;

For carbs (C) = 4 calories x 1g carb (since 1 gram of carbs gives 4 calories)

For proteins (P) = 4 calories x 1g protein (1 gram of protein also gives 4 calories)

The second step in the derivation of the CP formula considers an arbitrary metabolic index. Since they have normal metabolism and the ability to burn fat and induce thermogenesis, etc, proteins are assigned a metabolic index of 2, while carbs are assigned a metabolic index of 1. The metabolic index is then divided by the number of calories.

Therefore;

For carbs (C) = (4 calories x 1g carb) / 1

For protein (P) = (4 calories x 1g protein) / 2

The next step is to get the CP formula. To get the CP formula, simply divide (C) and (P) from above.

Therefore;

CP = [(4 calories x 1g carb) / 1] / [(4 calories x 1g protein) / 2]

Which simply amounts to CP = 2 x grams of carbs / grams of protein

The formula is not yet complete since it hasn't accounted for the fiber content of the carbs. The last step of the formula multiplies the number of grams of carbs by the fiber index.

Therefore;

CP = (2 x grams of carbs x fiber index) / grams of protein

Below are the assigned indices for fiber:

- Very high-fiber = 0.25
- High-fiber = 0.50
- Moderate fiber = 0.75
- Low or no fiber = 1.00

The fiber index is important since it accounts for the difference in absolute caloric contribution from carbs that are absorbed into the bloodstream and those that are not (fiber). It is even equally important for ensuring that high fiber foods are included in the diet. Some high-fiber foods have been shown to reduce the risk of cardiovascular disease and some cancers. High-fiber foods can also affect a modest weight loss.

What happens then to the formula when there is zero gram of protein or carb? 0 g is replaced with 0.0001g - the formula assumes a seasoning effect. The seasoning effect is simply the fact that very small (trace) amounts of protein or carb may be derived from the seasoning(s) used in cooking, and therefore the absolute amount of carbohydrate or protein is never zero. Adjusting for the seasoning effect is insignificant and inconsequential to the output of the CP formula.

The lower the CP value, the better the food is for weight loss. Foods with the lowest CP values have been placed in the 'green' table ('Green' Rotation One Table) and are ideal for rapid weight loss. Foods with moderately higher CP values have been placed in the 'yellow' table ('Yellow' Rotation One Table) and are ideal for slower weight loss and for weight maintenance when used together with foods in the 'green' table. During the weight loss phase, foods should be chosen from the 'green' and 'yellow' tables to make a balanced diet. The smaller the CP index, the better the food is for weight loss. Foods in the 'red' table ('Red' Rotation One Table) should be avoided.

■

Derivation of the FP formula

Like the CP formula, the first step in the derivation of the FP formula considers the number of calories provided by 1 gram of protein and 1 gram of fat. It starts by multiplying the number of calories to number of grams.

Therefore;

For fats (F) = 9 calories x 1g fat (since 1 gram of fat provides 9 calories)

For proteins (P) = 4 calories x 1g protein (1 gram of protein provides 4 calories)

The second step in the derivation of the CP formula considers an arbitrary metabolic index. Since they have normal metabolism and the ability to burn fat and induce thermogenesis, etc, proteins are assigned a metabolic index of 2, while carbs are assigned a metabolic index of 1. The metabolic index is then divided by the number of calories.

Therefore;

For fats (F) = (9 calories x 1g fat) / 1

For protein (P) = (4 calories x 1g protein) / 2

The next step is to get the FP formula. To get the FP formula simply divide (F) and (P) from above.

Therefore;

FP = [(9 calories x 1g fat) / 1] / [(4 calories x 1g protein) / 2]

Which simply amounts to FP = 4.5 x grams of fat / grams of protein

It is unnecessary to adjust for fiber in this case, since we are tagging fats (not carbohydrates) to protein.

Therefore;

$$FP = (4.5 \times \text{grams of fats}) / \text{grams of protein}$$

As was the case with the CP formula, the FP formula assumes the seasoning effect and replaces 0 g fat or 0 g protein with 0.0001g. Adjusting for the seasoning effect is insignificant and inconsequential to the output of the FP formula.

The lower the FP value, the better the food is for weight loss. Foods with the lowest FP values have been placed in the 'green' table ('Green' Rotation Two Table) and are ideal for rapid weight loss. Foods with moderately higher FP values have been placed in the 'yellow' table ('Yellow' Rotation Two Table) and are ideal for weight maintenance when used together with foods in the 'green' table. During the weight loss phase, foods should be chosen from the 'green' and 'yellow' tables to make a balanced diet. The smaller the FP index, the better the food is for weight loss. Foods in the 'red' table ('Red' Rotation Two Table) should be avoided.

How cutoff values of CP and FP were determined

The cutoff values of CP and FP are based on standardizing against the recommended diet of a healthy, non-obese adult (25 year old) human. If all the recommended amounts of carbs, fats and proteins of a healthy, non-obese adult were pooled together as one meal, the CP value for that meal will be approximately 12.0 and the FP value will be approximately 5.9.

The cutoff values of CP and FP for the plateau-proof diets are significantly below these values in the 'green' tables, and slightly below these values in the 'yellow' tables. Since obesity is a chronic condition, CP and FP values have to remain at relatively lower values even after complete weight loss has been attained. It is therefore highly recommended that during the maintenance phase (after desired weight loss has been achieved) foods should still be chosen from both the 'green' and the 'yellow' tables, while the 'red' tables should be avoided as much as possible.

The CP cutoff values are 2.0 for the 'Green' table and 10.0 for the 'Yellow' table. The FP cutoff values are 1.0 for the 'Green' table and 3.0 for the 'Yellow' table.

How to use the plateau-proof diet

1) Start the diet with the CP 'Green' and 'Yellow' Tables. Make balanced meals out of the food items in these tables. Eat as wide a variety of foods as you are able to. Do this for 4 weeks. Avoid items in the 'Red' table. *[Note: if you are just getting off a low-carb diet program (within 2 weeks), start the plateau-proof diet with FP 'Green' and 'Yellow' tables.]*

2) At the end of 4 weeks, eat foods from the FP 'Green' and 'Yellow' tables for 2 weeks. Eat the widest variety of foods possible. Avoid foods in the 'Red' table. You probably are going to be at the peak of your weight loss from the CP rotation when you start the FP rotation. Once you are in the FP rotation, your rate of weight loss may be significantly lower than it was on the CP rotation. You should however complete this 2 week rotation before going back to the CP rotation. Remember that this is the strategy for avoiding the dreaded weight loss plateau. *Always try to balance your meals, and avoid eating the same items repeatedly.*

3) At the end of one week, go back to the CP rotation and keep alternating until you achieve complete weight loss. *Keep a daily record of the food items you eat and your weight.* When you achieve your desired weight loss, continue the diet with fewer restrictions to maintain your new lean body.

How much food should you eat?

There are many factors that determine how much food is required by your body each day. These factors include lean body mass and level of activity. Since no two people are identical in this regard, it is impractical to assign a fixed quantity of food for everyone. A more practical approach for the plateau-proof diet is that you start the diet by cutting down your normal portion modestly. It would be beneficial to start by cutting down about 10 – 20 % of your original portion in the first rotation (4 weeks). You should then cut down an additional 5 – 10 % during each subsequent rotation. The minimum daily amount of food that you should eat after cutting down the portion size should be approximately 400 grams (14.1 ounces). You may not experience a robust weight loss until your daily food intake approaches the recommended daily minimum; however, your cardiovascular risk factors should improve from the beginning. When it comes to portion size, it is more important to start slowly and finish strongly, than to start strongly and never finish. In other words, it may be more beneficial to set your mentality for a marathon rather than a sprint.

If you believe that the cause of your weight problem is overeating and you are unable to sustain a portion restricting diet, please seek immediate help from your health care provider.

When should you eat?

It doesn't matter when you eat. You can eat at any time. Some studies have suggested that people who eat breakfast tend to lose weight better than people who don't eat breakfast. Also, it is better to eat your meals in many small portions throughout the day as opposed to one large portion.

The plateau-proof diet and prepackaged foods

You can evaluate prepackaged foods on an individual bases for compliance with the plateau-proof diet guidelines. Avoid prepackaged foods that contain trans fats and those that are high in sodium (salt).

1) *Evaluating a food for the CP rotation*
To evaluate a prepackaged food for the CP rotation, read its nutrition label and enter the amount of protein, carbohydrate, and fiber into the CP formula:

> *CP = (2 x grams of carbs x fiber index) / grams of protein*

Convert grams of fiber into the fiber index using the table below:

Fiber content	Fiber index
- Very high-fiber (≥ 10 g per serving)	= 0.25
- High-fiber (≥ 5 g per serving)	= 0.50
- Moderate fiber(≥ 1 g per serving)	= 0.75
- Low or no fiber (< 1 g per serving)	= 1.00

If the CP value is equal to or less than 2.0, the prepackaged food is a CP 'Green' table food. If the CP value is equal to or less than 10.0 but greater than 2.0, the prepackaged food belongs in the CP 'Yellow' table. In either case, this food can be eaten during the 4 week CP rotation. If the CP value is greater than 10.0, the food cannot be eaten during the 4 week CP rotation.

2) *Evaluating a food for the FP rotation*

To evaluate a prepackaged food for the FP rotation, read its nutrition label and enter the amount of protein and total fat into the FP formula:

$$FP = (4.5 \times grams\ of\ fats) / grams\ of\ protein$$

If the FP value is equal to or less than 1.0, the food belongs in the FP 'Green' table and can be eaten during the 2 week FP rotation. If the FP value is equal to or less than 3.0 but greater than 1.0, the food belongs in the FP 'Yellow' table and can be eaten during the 2 week FP rotation. If the food has an FP value greater than 3.0, it cannot be eaten during the 2 week FP rotation.

Please note:

(1) If a prepackaged food contains trans fats it should be avoided regardless of its CP or FP values.

(2) The plateau-proof diet cardio (next chapter) separates saturated fats (not good for your cardiovascular health) from total fats. The formula for evaluating prepackaged foods is therefore different for the plateau-proof diet cardio. The plateau-proof diet cardio is the healthier heart version of the plateau-proof diet, and I highly recommend it over the plateau-proof diet.

CP 'GREEN' TABLE

Eat foods from this table for 4 weeks along with foods from the CP 'Yellow' table.

Name of food	CP value
ALFALFA SEEDS (SPROUTED, RAW)	1.5
ALMONDS (SLIVERED)	1.6
AMERICAN CHEESE	0.0
AMERICAN CHEESE SPREAD	0.8
ASPARAGUS (FROZEN)	1.5
BEANS (CANNED, FRANKFURTER)	1.7
BEEF (DRIED)	0.0
BEEF (LEAN & FAT CHUCK BLADE)	0.0
BEEF (LEAN & FAT, BOTTOM ROUND)	0.0
BEEF (LEAN, BOTTOM ROUND)	0.0
BEEF (LEAN, CHUCK BLADE)	0.0
BEEF AND VEGETABLE STEW	1.4
BEEF BROTH (BOULLION)	0.0
BEEF HEART (BRAISED)	0.0
BEEF LIVER (FRIED)	0.6
BEEF ROAST (LEAN, EYE O RND)	0.0
BEEF ROAST (LEAN & FAT, EYE O RND)	0.0
BEEF ROAST (LEAN & FAT, RIBS)	0.0
BEEF ROAST (LEAN, RIBS)	0.0
BEEF STEAK (LEAN, SIRLOIN, BROIL)	0.0
BLACK BEANS (COOKED, DRAINED)	1.4
BLACK-EYED PEAS, DRY, COOKED	1.5
BLUE CHEESE	0.3
BOLOGNA	0.6
BRAUNSCHWEIGER	0.5

BRAZIL NUTS	1.5
BROCCOLI (FROZEN, COOKED, DRAINED)	1.7
BUTTER	0.0
CABBAGE (CHINESE)	1.5
CAMEMBERT CHEESE	0.0
CHEDDAR CHEESE	0.0
CHICKEN (CANNED)	0.0
CHICKEN (LIGHT & DARK, STEWED)	0.0
CHICKEN A LA KING	0.9
CHICKEN BREAST (FRIED, BATTERED)	0.7
CHICKEN BREAST (FRIED, FLOUR)	0.1
CHICKEN BREAST (ROASTED)	0.0
CHICKEN DRUMSTICK (FRIED, BATTERED)	0.8
CHICKEN DRUMSTICK (ROASTED)	0.0
CHICKEN DRUMSTICK, (FRIED, FLOUR)	0.2
CHICKEN FRANKFURTER	1.0
CHICKEN LIVER	0.0
CHICKEN ROLL	0.2
CHOP SUEY (BEEF & PORK)	1.0
CLAMS	0.4
CORNED BEEF (CANNED)	0.0
COTTAGE CHEESE (LARGE CURDS, CREAMED)	0.4
COTTAGE CHEESE (LOWFAT 2%)	0.5
COTTAGE CHEESE (UNCREAMED)	0.2
CRABMEAT	0.1
CREAM CHEESE	1.0
DUCK (ROASTED)	0.0
EGGS (FRIED)	0.3
EGGS (HARD-BOILED)	0.3
EGGS (POACHED)	0.3

EGGS (SCRAMBLED)	0.3
EGGS (WHITE, RAW)	0.0
EGGS (WHOLE, RAW)	0.3
EGGS (YOLK, RAW)	0.0
FETA CHEESE	0.5
FISH STICKS	1.3
FLOUNDER (BAKED IN BUTTER)	0.0
FLOUNDER (BAKED IN MARGARINE)	0.0
FLOUNDER (BAKED, NO FAT)	0.0
FRANKFURTER	0.4
GROUND BEEF (BROILED, LEAN & FAT)	0.0
GROUND BEEF (BROILED, LEAN)	0.0
HADDOCK (BREADED, FRIED)	0.8
HALIBUT (BROILED, BUTTER & LEMON JUICE)	0.0
HERRING (PICKLED)	0.0
LAMB (LEG, LEAN & FAT, ROASTED)	0.0
LAMB (LEG, LEAN, ROASTED)	0.0
LAMB CHOPS (ARM, LEAN & FAT, BRAISED)	0.0
LAMB CHOPS (ARM, LEAN, BRAISED)	0.0
LAMB CHOPS (LOIN, LEAN & FAT, BROIL)	0.0
LAMB CHOPS (LOIN, LEAN, BROIL)	0.0
LAMB RIB (LEAN & FAT, ROASTED)	0.0
LAMB RIB (LEAN, ROASTED)	0.0
LENTILS	1.2
MIXED NUTS (OIL ROASTED, NO HONEY)	1.8
MOZZARELLA CHEESE (WHOLE MILK)	0.3
MOZZARELLA CHESE (SKIM MILK)	0.3
MUENSTER CHEESE	0.0
OCEAN PERCH (FRIED, BREADED)	0.9

OYSTERS (RAW)	0.8
PARMESAN CHEESE	0.2
PEANUT BUTTER	1.2
PEANUTS (OIL-ROASTED)	1.3
PISTACHIO NUTS	1.8
PORK (CURED, BACON)	0.0
PORK (CURED, CANADIAN BACON)	0.2
PORK (CURED, HAM, LEAN & FAT)	0.0
PORK (CURED, HAM, LEAN)	0.0
PORK (LINK)	0.0
PORK (LUNCHEON MEAT, CANNED)	0.4
PORK (LUNCHEON MEAT, HAM, LEAN & FAT)	0.4
PORK (LUNCHEON MEAT, HAM, LEAN)	0.2
PORK (ROASTED HAM, LEAN)	0.0
PORK CHOP LOIN (BROILED, LEAN & FAT)	0.0
PORK CHOP LOIN (BROILED, LEAN)	0.0
PORK CHOP LOIN (FRIED, LEAN & FAT)	0.0
PORK CHOP LOIN (FRIED, LEAN)	0.0
PORK FRESH (ROASTED HAM, LEAN & FAT)	0.0
PORK RIBS (ROASTED, LEAN & FAT)	0.0
PORK RIBS (ROASTED, LEAN)	0.0
PORK SHOULDER (BRAISED, LEAN & FAT)	0.0
PORK SHOULDER (BRAISED, LEAN)	0.0
PROVOLONE CHEESE	0.3
PUMPKIN AND SQUASH KERNELS	1.4
RICOTTA CHEESE (SKIM MILK)	0.9
RICOTTA CHEESE (WHOLE MILK)	0.5
SALAMI (DRY)	0.4
SALAMI (NOT DRY)	0.3
SALMON (CANNED)	0.0

SALMON (RED, BAKED)	0.0
SALMON (SMOKED)	0.0
SARDINES (CANNED, OIL, ATLANTIC)	0.0
SAUSAGE (BROWN AND SERVE)	0.0
SCALLOPS (BREADED)	1.3
SEAWEED (SPIRULINA)	0.9
SESAME SEEDS	1.0
SHRIMP	0.1
SHRIMP (FRIED, NOT BREADED, NOT BATTERED)	1.4
SOLE (BAKED IN MARGARINE)	0.0
SOLE (BAKED IN BUTTER)	0.0
SOLE (BAKED, NO FAT)	0.0
SOYBEANS	1.5
SPINACH (CANNED)	1.8
SPINACH (FRESH)	1.5
SPINACH SOUFFLE	0.5
STEAK (BROILED, SIRLOIN)	0.0
SUNFLOWER SEEDS	1.7
SWISS CHEESE	0.3
PARMESAN CHEESE	0.2
TOFU	0.7
TROUT (BROILED, BUTTER)	0.0
TUNA (CANNED, LIGHT, OIL, DRAINNED)	0.0
TUNA (CANNED, LIGHT, WATER)	0.0
TUNA SALAD	1.2
TURKEY (LIGHT & DARK, ROASTED)	0.0
TURKEY (ROASTED)	0.0
TURKEY HAM (CURED)	0.0
TURKEY LOAF	0.0
VEAL CUTLET (BROILED, ROASTED,	0.0

BRAISED)	
VEAL RIB (BROILED, ROASTED, BRAISED)	0.0
VIENNA SAUSAGE	0.0
WALNUTS (BLACK)	0.6
WALNUTS (ENGLISH)	1.9

CP 'YELLOW' TABLE

Eat foods from this table for 4 weeks along with foods from the CP 'Green' table.

Name of food	CP value
ALL-BRAN CEREAL	5.3
ARTICHOKES (GLOBE, COOKED)	6.0
ASPARAGUS (CANNED)	3.0
AVOCADOS (CALIFORNIA)	6.0
BAMBOO SHOOTS (CANNED)	3.0
BEAN SPROUTS	2.5
BEAN WITH BACON SOUP	2.9
BEANS (PORK, SWEET SAUCE)	3.4
BEANS (PORK, TOMATO SAUCE)	3.0
BEEF GRAVY	2.4
BEEF NOODLE SOUP	3.6
BEEF POTPIE	3.7
BEER (LIGHT)	10.0
BEET GREENS	3.0
BLUE CHEESE SALAD DRESSING	2.0
BOUILLON (DEHYDRATED)	2.0
BROCCOLI (RAW, COOKED, DRAINED)	2.3
BROWN GRAVY (DRY MIX)	9.3
BRUSSELS SPROUTS	3.3
BUTTERMILK (DRIED)	2.9
BUTTERMILK (LIQUID)	3.4
CABBAGE (RED)	6.0
CABBAGE (SAVOY)	6.0
CANDY (MILK CHOCOLATE, ALMONDS)	10.0

CANDY (MILK CHOCOLATE, PEANUTS)	6.5
CARROTS (FROZEN, COOKED)	9.0
CASHEW NUTS (DRY ROASTD)	4.5
CASHEW NUTS (ROASTED, OIL)	3.5
CAULIFLOWER	4.5
CELERY (PASCAL, RAW)	2.0
CELERY SEED	10.0
CEREAL (100% NATURAL)	6.0
CHEERIOS CEREAL	10.0
CHEESE CRACKERS (PEANUT SANDWICH)	10.0
CHEESE SAUCE WITH MILK	2.9
CHEESEBURGER	3.7
CHICKEN AND NOODLES	2.4
CHICKEN CHOW MEIN	5.1
CHICKEN GRAVY (CANNED)	5.2
CHICKEN GRAVY (DRY MIX)	9.3
CHICKEN NOODLE SOUP	4.5
CHICKEN POTPIE	3.8
CHICKEN RICE SOUP	3.5
CHICKPEAS	3.2
CHILI	2.4
CHOCOLATE (FOR BAKING, BITTER)	5.3
CHOCOLATE MILK (LOWFAT 1%)	6.5
CHOCOLATE MILK (LOWFAT 2%)	6.5
CHOCOLATE MILK (REGULAR)	6.5
CHOW MEIN NOODLES	8.7
CLAM CHOWDER (MANHATTAN)	6.0
CLAM CHOWDER (NEW ENGLAND, MILK)	3.8
CLUB SODA	2.0
COCOA POWDER (REGULAR)	6.7
COFFEE	2.0

COFFEE CREAM (LIGHT)	3.0
COLA (DIET)	2.0
COLLARDS	3.8
CORN (RAW, WHITE)	9.5
CORN OIL	2.0
COTTAGE CHEESE (FRUIT)	2.9
CREAM OF CHICKEN SOUP (MILK)	4.3
CREAM OF CHICKEN SOUP (WATER)	6.0
CREAM OF MUSHROM SOUP (MILK)	5.0
CREAM OF MUSHROOM SOUP (WATER)	9.0
CUSTARD (BAKED)	4.5
CUSTARD PIE	8.2
DANDELION GREENS	5.3
EGG NOG	7.6
ENCHILADA	2.4
ENDIVE	4.0
ENG MUFFIN (BACON, EGG, CHEESE)	3.4
EVAPORATED MILK (SKIM)	3.1
EVAPORATED MILK (WHOLE)	2.9
FILBERTS (HAZELNUTS)	2.4
FISH SANDWICH (CHEESE)	4.9
FISH SANDWICH (NO CHEESE)	4.6
GREAT NORTHERN BEANS (DRY, DRAINED)	2.9
GREEN PEAS (SOUP)	4.5
HALF AND HALF (CREAM)	2.9
HOLLANDAISE (WATER)	5.6
ICE MILK (VANILLA, 3%)	9.5
IMITATION SOUR DRESSING	2.8
KALE	3.5
KOHLRABI	7.3
LEMONS (RAW)	10.0

LETTUCE (BUTTER-HEAD)	4.0
LETTUCE (CRISP-HEAD)	4.4
LETTUCE (LOOSE LEAF)	4.0
LIMA BEANS	3.1
LIQUOR (GIN, RUM, VODKA, WHISKY, COGNAC...)	2.0
MACADAMIA NUTS (OIL ROASTED)	3.4
MACARONI AND CHEESE	4.7
MALTED MILK (CHOCOLATE)	6.4
MALTED MILK (REGULAR)	4.9
MARGARINE (REGULAR, HARD)	2.0
MARGARINE (IMITATION 40% FAT)	2.0
MARGARINE (REGULAR, HARD, 80% FAT)	2.0
MARGARINE (REGULR, SOFT)	2.0
MARGARINE (REGULR, SOFT, 80% FAT)	2.0
MARGARINE (SPREAD, HARD, 60% FAT)	2.0
MARGARINE (SPREAD, SOFT, 60% FAT)	2.0
MAYONNAISE (REGULAR)	2.0
MELBA TOAST	8.0
MILK (1% LOW FAT)	2.7
MILK (2% LOW FAT)	2.7
MILK (NONFAT)	2.7
MILK (WHOLE)	2.8
MINESTRONE SOUP	5.5
MISO	4.6
MIXED GRAIN BREAD	9.4
MIXED NUTS (DRY ROASTED, NO HONEY)	2.6
MUSHROOM GRAVY	8.7
MUSHROOMS (CANNED)	5.3
MUSHROOMS (RAW)	6.0
MUSTARD (YELLOW)	2.0

MUSTARD GREENS	2.0
NONFAT DRY MILK	3.0
OATMEAL (PLAIN)	9.0
OKRA	4.5
OLIVE OIL	2.0
OLIVES (BLACK)	2.0
OLIVES (GREEN)	2.0
ONION SOUP	8.0
ONIONS (RAW, SPRING)	4.0
OYSTERS (FRIED, BREADED)	2.0
PEA BEANS (DRY)	4.0
PEANUT OIL	2.0
PEAS (CANNED, GREEN)	5.3
PEAS (FRESH, GREEN)	4.3
PEAS (POD)	3.3
PECANS (HALVES)	5.0
PEPPERS (HOT GREEN CHILI)	8.0
PEPPERS (HOT RED CHILI)	8.0
PEPPERS (SWEET GREEN)	8.0
PEPPERS (SWEET RED)	8.0
PINE NUTS	5.0
PINTO BEANS	4.9
PIZZA (CHEESE)	5.6
POPCORN (AIR-POPPED)	9.0
POPCORN (VEGETABLE OIL)	9.0
POTATO SALAD (MAYONNAISE)	8.0
QUICHE LORRAINE	4.5
RED KIDNEY BEANS	2.8
REFRIED BEANS	4.3
ROAST BEEF SANDWICH	3.1
RYE BREAD (LIGHT)	8.6

SAFFLOWER OIL	2.0
SANDWICH SPREAD (BEEF & PORK)	4.0
SAUERKRAUT	7.5
SNAP BEAN (GREEN)	4.5
SNAP BEAN (YELLOW)	4.5
SOUR CREAM	2.9
SOY SAUCE	2.0
SOYBEAN OIL	2.0
SOYBEAN-COTTONSEED OIL	2.0
SPAGHETTI (FIRM)	8.4
SPAGHETTI (MEATBALLS, TOMATO SAUCE)	4.8
SPECIAL K CEREAL	7.0
SPINACH (FROZEN)	2.5
SQUASH (SUMMER)	8.0
SUNFLOWER OIL	2.0
TACO	3.3
TAHINI	2.0
TEA (BREWED, UNSWEETENED)	2.0
TOMATO JUICE	10.0
TOMATO SOUP (MILK)	7.3
TOMATOES (CANNED)	10.0
TOMATOES (FRESH)	7.5
TORTILLAS (CORN)	9.8
TURKEY AND GRAVY	2.0
TURKEY PATTIES (BATTERED, FRIED)	2.2
TURNIP GREENS (FRESH)	6.0
TURNIP GREENS (FROZEN)	3.2
VEGETABLE & BEEF SOUP	2.5
VEGETABLE JUICE	8.3
VEGETABLES (MIXED)	5.6
VEGETARIAN SOUP	9.0

VINEGAR AND OIL SALAD DRESSING	**2.0**
WAFFLES	**7.7**
WHEAT CRACKERS	**10.0**
WHIPPED TOPPING	**7.0**
WHIPPING CREAM (HEAVY)	**2.8**
WHIPPING CREAM (LIGHT)	**2.8**
WHITE SAUCE (MILK)	**4.2**
WHOLE-WHEAT BREAD	**7.2**
WHOLE-WHEAT FLOUR	**8.0**
WHOLE-WHEAT WAFERS	**7.5**
YOGURT (FRUIT, LOW FAT MILK)	**8.6**
YOGURT (NONFAT MILK)	**2.8**
YOGURT (PLAIN, LOW FAT MILK)	**2.7**
YOGURT (WHOLE MILK)	**2.8**

CP 'RED' TABLE

Avoid the foods in this table during this 4 week rotation.

Name of food	CP value
ANGELFOOD CAKE	18.0
APPLE JUICE (CANNED)	58000.0
APPLE PIE	34.3
APPLE PIE (FRIED)	31.0
APPLES (RAW, UNPEELED)	480.0
APPLES (DRIED, SULFURED)	630.0
APPLESAUCE (CANNED, SWEETENED)	1020.0
APPLESAUCE (CANNED,UNSWEETENED)	560.0
APRICOT (CANNED, HEAVY SYRUP)	110.0
APRICOT NECTAR	72.0
APRICOTS (CANNED, IN JUICE)	31.0
APRICOTS (DRIED)	27.5
APRICOTS (RAW)	18.0
AVOCADOS (FLORIDA)	10.8
BAGELS (EGG)	10.9
BAGELS (PLAIN)	10.9
BANANAS	54.0
BARBECUE SAUCE	4000.0
BARLEY (PEARLED, LIGHT)	14.8
BEER (REGULAR)	26.0
BEETS (CANNED)	12.0
BEETS (COOKED, DRAINED)	14.0
BISCUIT BAKING MIX	14.0
BLACKBERRIES (RAW)	27.0
BLUEBERRIES (FROZEN, SWEETENED)	100.0
BLUEBERRIES (RAW)	40.0
BLUEBERRY MUFFINS	13.3

BLUEBERRY PIE	28.7
BOSTON BROWN BREAD	21.0
BRAN FLAKES (40%)	11.0
BRAN MUFFINS	12.0
BREAD STUFFING (DRY MIX)	11.1
BREADCRUMBS	11.2
BROWNIES WITH NUTS	22.0
BUCKWHEAT FLOUR (LIGHT, SIFTED)	19.5
BULGUR	13.6
CABBAGE (COMMON)	10.5
CAKE & PASTRY FLOUR	21.7
CANDY (MILK CHOCOLATE, PLAIN)	16.0
CANDY (MILK CHOCOLATE, RICE CRISPIES)	18.0
CANTALOUP	22.0
CAP'N CRUNCH CEREAL	46.0
CARAMEL	44.0
CAROB FLOUR	42.0
CARROT CAKE (CREME CHESE FROSTING)	24.6
CARROTS (RAW)	12.0
CATSUP	27.6
CHEESE CRACKERS (PLAIN)	12.0
CHEESECAKE	11.3
CHERRIES (RAW, SWEET)	22.0
CHERRIES (SOUR, CANNED, WATER)	44.0
CHERRY PIE	29.0
CHERRY PIE (FRIED)	32.0
CHESTNUTS (ROASTED)	30.4
CHOCOLATE (SWEET, DARK)	32.0
CHOCOLATE CHIP COOKIES	28.0
CHOCOLATE PUDDING	13.5

CHOCOLATE SHAKE	15.0
COCOA POWDER (NO FAT DRY MILK)	14.7
COCONUT (RAW)	10.5
COCONUT (SHREDDED, DRIED, SWEETENED)	22.0
COFFEECAKE (CRUMB)	16.7
COLA (REGULAR)	82000.0
CONDENSED MILK (SWEETENED)	13.8
CORN (CREAM, CANNED)	23.0
CORN (RAW, YELLOW)	14.3
CORN CHIPS	16.0
CORN FLAKES	24.0
CORN GRITS (WHITE)	20.7
CORN GRITS (YELLOW)	20.7
CORN MUFFINS	14.0
CORNMEAL	16.4
CRACKED-WHEAT BREAD	12.0
CRACKED-WHEAT BREAD	10.8
CRACKERS (SNACK)	40.0
CRANBERRY JUICE COCKTAL	76000.0
CRANBERRY SAUCE (SWEATENED, CANNED)	216.0
CREAM OF WHEAT	14.0
CREME PIE	35.1
CROISSANTS	10.8
CUCUMBER (WITH PEEL)	200.0
DANISH PASTRY (FRUIT)	14.0
DANISH PASTRY (PLAIN)	14.5
DATES	32.8
DEVIL'S FOOD CAKE (CHOCOLATE FROSTING)	28.7

DOUGHNUTS (CAKE TYPE, PLAIN)	16.0
DOUGHNUTS (YEAST-LEAVENED, GLAZED)	17.3
EGG NOODLES	10.6
EGGPLANT	12.0
ENGLISH MUFFINS (PLAIN)	10.8
FIG BARS	31.5
FIGS (DRIED)	20.3
FRENCH BREAD	10.7
FRENCH SALAD DRESSING (LOW CAL)	4000.0
FRENCH SALAD DRESSING (REGULAR)	2000.0
FROOT LOOPS CEREAL	25.0
FROSTED FLAKES CEREAL	52.0
FRUIT COCKTAIL (CANNED, HEAVY SYRUP)	96.0
FRUIT COCKTAIL (CANNED, JUICE)	58.0
FRUIT JELLIES	20000.0
FRUIT PUNCH DRINK (CANNED)	44000.0
FRUITCAKE	21.2
FUDGE, CHOCOLATE, PLAIN	42.0
GELATIN DESSERT	17.0
GINGER ALE	64000.0
GINGERBREAD CAKE	32.3
GOLDEN GRAHAMS CEREAL	24.0
GRAHAM CRACKER (PLAIN)	22.0
GRAPE DRINK (CANNED)	52000.0
GRAPE JUICE (CANNED)	76.0
GRAPE SODA	92000.0
GRAPEFRUIT (CANNED, SYRUP)	78.0
GRAPEFRUIT (RAW)	20.0
GRAPEFRUIT JUICE (SWEETENED)	56.0
GRAPEFRUIT JUICE (UNSWEETENED)	48.0

GRAPE-NUTS CEREAL	15.3
GRAPES (RAW)	1800.0
GUM DROPS	50000.0
HARD CANDY	56000.0
HONEY	558.0
HONEY NUT CHEERIOS CEREAL	15.3
HONEYDEW MELON	24.0
ICE CREAM (VANLLA,11% FAT)	13.4
ICE CREAM (VANLLA,16% FAT)	15.5
ICE MILK (VANILLA, 4% FAT)	11.3
IMITATION CREAMER (POWDERED)	2000.0
IMITATION WHIPPED TOPING	2000.0
ITALIAN BREAD	12.8
ITALIAN SALAD DRESSING (LOW CAL)	400.0
ITALIAN SALAD DRESSING (REGULAR)	200.0
JAMS AND FRUIT PRESERVES	20000.0
JELLY BEANS	52000.0
JERUSALEM-ARTICHOKE	13.0
KIWIFRUIT	22.0
LEMON JUICE	32.0
LEMON MERINGUE PIE	20.5
LEMONADE	42000.0
LEMON-LIME SODA	78000.0
LUCKY CHARMS CEREAL	15.3
MACARONI	11.1
MALT-O-MEAL	13.0
MANGO (RAW)	70.0
MARSHMALLOWS	46.0
MAYONNAISE (IMITATION)	4000.0
MAYONNAISE SALAD DRESSING	8000.0
MOLASSES	44000.0

NATURE VALLEY GRANOLA CEREAL	12.7
NECTARINES	32.0
OATMEAL & RAISIN COOKIES	24.0
OATMEAL (FLAVORED)	12.4
OATMEAL BREAD	11.2
ONION RINGS	16.0
ONIONS (RAW)	12.0
ORANGE & GRAPEFRUIT JUICE	50.0
ORANGE (RAW)	30.0
ORANGE JUICE (CANNED)	50.0
ORANGE JUICE (FRESH)	26.0
ORANGE SODA	92000.0
PANCAKES (BUCKWHEAT)	12.0
PANCAKES (PLAIN)	16.0
PAPAYA	34.0
PARSNIPS	22.5
PEACH PIE	30.1
PEACHES (CANNED, HEAVY SYRUP)	102.0
PEACHES (CANNED, JUICE)	29.0
PEACHES (DRIED)	32.7
PEACHES (FRESH)	20.0
PEANUT BUTTER COOKIE	14.0
PEAR (CANNED, HEAVY SYRUP)	98.0
PEAR (CANNED, JUICE)	64.0
PEAR (FRESH)	37.5
PECAN PIE	20.1
PICKLES (CUCUMBER)	600.0
PICKLES (CUCUMBER, DILL)	200.0
PICKLES (CUCUMBER, SWEET)	1000.0
PIE CRUST	14.1
PINEAPPLE (CANNED, HEAVY SYRUP)	104.0

PINEAPPLE (CANNED, JUICE)	78.0
PINEAPPLE (FRESH)	38.0
PINEAPPLE JUICE (UNSWEETENED)	68.0
PINEAPPLE-GRAPEFRUIT JUICE DRINK	46000.0
PITA BREAD	11.0
PLANTAINS	42.8
PLUMS (CANNED, HEAVY SYRUP)	120.0
PLUMS (CANNED, JUICE)	76.0
PLUMS (FRESH)	18.0
POPCORN (SYRUP)	22.5
POPSICLE	36000.0
POTATO CHIPS	20.0
POTATOES (AU GRATIN)	12.4
POTATOES (BAKED, NO SKIN)	22.7
POTATOES (BAKED, WITH SKIN)	20.4
POTATOES (BOILED)	18.0
POTATOES (FRENCH FRIES, BAKED)	17.0
POTATOES (FRENCH FRIES, FRIED)	20.0
POTATOES (HASHED BROWN)	17.6
POTATOES (MASHED)	16.0
POTATOES (SCALLOPED)	12.4
POUND CAKE	19.8
PRETZELS	13.0
PRODUCT 19 CEREAL	16.0
PRUNE JUICE	22.5
PRUNES (DRIED)	31.0
PUMPERNICKEL BREAD	10.6
PUMPKIN (CANNED)	13.3
PUMPKIN (FRESH)	12.0
PUMPKIN PIE	12.7
RADISHES	200.0

RAISIN BRAN CEREAL	10.5
RAISIN BREAD	13.0
RAISINS	34.5
RASPBERRIES (SWEETENED)	55.5
RELISH (SWEET)	100.0
RHUBARB (SWEETENED)	150.0
RICE (BROWN)	20.0
RICE (WHITE)	25.0
RICE KRISPIES CEREAL	25.0
RICE PUDDING	13.5
ROLLS (DINNER)	28.0
ROLLS (FRANKFURTER & HAMBURGER)	13.3
ROLLS (HARD)	12.0
ROLLS (HOAGIE OR SUBMARINE)	13.1
ROOT BEER	84000.0
RYE WAFERS (WHOLE-GRAIN)	15.0
SALTINES	18.0
SEAWEED (KELP)	60.0
SELF-RISING FLOUR (UNSIFTED)	15.5
SEMI SWEET CHOCOLATE	27.7
SHEETCAKE (NO FROSTING)	26.3
SHEETCAKE (WHITE FROSTING)	51.3
SHERBET	55.2
SHORTBREAD COOKIE	20.0
SHREDDED WHEAT CEREAL	11.5
SNACK CAKES (DEVIL'S FOOD & CRÈME)	34.0
SNACK CAKES (SPONGE & CRÈME)	54.0
SPAGHETTI (SOFT)	12.8
SPAGHETTI (TOMATO SAUCE, CHEESE)	13.0
SQUASH (WINTER)	18.0
STRAWBERRIES (FRESH)	15.0

STRAWBERRIES (FROZEN, SWEETENED)	55.5
SUGAR (BROWN)	424000.0
SUGAR (WHITE)	398000.0
SUGAR COOKIE	31.0
SUGAR SMACKS CEREAL	25.0
SUPER SUGAR CRISP CEREAL	26.0
SWEET POTATOE PIE	58000.0
SWEET POTATOES (BAKED)	21.0
SWEETPOTATOES (CANNED)	12.0
SWEETPOTATOES (CANNED, MASHED)	23.6
SYRUP (LIGHT, CHOCOLATE FLAVORED)	44.0
SYRUP (CORN, MAPLE)	64000.0
SYRUP (THICK, CHOCOLATE FLAVORED)	21.0
TANGERINE JUICE	60.0
TANGERINES (CANNED, LIGHT SYRUP)	82.0
TANGERINES (FRESH)	18.0
TAPIOCA PUDDING	18.7
TARTAR SAUCE	200.0
THOUSAND ISLAND DRESSING	400.0
TOASTER PASTRIES	38.0
TOMATO & VEGETABLE SOUP	12.0
TOMATO PASTE	10.9
TOMATO PUREE	12.5
TOMATO SOUP (WATER)	17.0
TOTAL CEREAL	14.7
TRIX CEREAL	25.0
TURNIPS	16.0
VANILLA PUDDING	33.0
VANILLA WAFERS	29.0
VIENNA BREAD	13.0
WATER CHESTNUTS	34.0

WATERMELON	23.3
WHEAT BREAD	10.1
WHEAT FLOUR (ALL-PURPOSE, SIFTED	14.7
WHEAT FLOUR (ALL-PURPOSE, UNSIFTED)	14.6
WHEATIES CEREAL	15.3
WHITE BREAD	12.0
WHITE BREAD CRUMBS	11.0
WHITE BREAD CUBES	15.0
WHITE CAKE (WHITE FROSTING)	31.2
YELLOW CAKE (CHOCOLATE FROSTING)	29.0

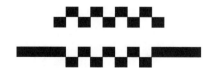

FP 'GREEN' TABLE

Eat foods from this table for 2 weeks along with foods from the FP 'Yellow' table.

Name of food	FP value
ALFALFA SEEDS (SPROUTED, RAW)	0.0
ANGELFOOD CAKE	0.2
APPLES (DRIED, SULFURED)	0.0
APRICOT (CANNED, HEAVY SYRUP)	0.0
APRICOT NECTAR	0.0
APRICOTS (CANNED, IN JUICE)	0.0
APRICOTS (DRIED)	0.0
APRICOTS (RAW)	0.0
ARTICHOKES (GLOBE, COOKED)	0.0
ASPARAGUS (CANNED)	0.0
ASPARAGUS (FROZEN)	0.0
BARLEY (PEARLED, LIGHT)	0.6
BEAN SPROUTS	0.0
BEEF (LEAN, DRIED)	0.8
BEEF HEART (BRAISED)	0.9
BEET GREENS	0.0
BEETS (CANNED)	0.0
BEETS (COOKED, DRAINED)	0.0
BLACK BEANS (COOKED, DRAINED)	0.3
BLACK-EYED PEAS, DRY, COOKED	0.4
BLUEBERRIES (FROZEN, SWEETENED)	0.0
BRAN FLAKES (40%)	0.0
BROCCOLI (FROZEN, COOKED, DRAINED)	0.0
BROCCOLI (RAW, COOKED, DRAINED)	0.0

BRUSSELS SPROUTS	0.8
BUCKWHEAT FLOUR (LIGHT, SIFTED)	0.8
BULGUR	0.7
CABBAGE (CHINESE)	0.0
CABBAGE (COMMON)	0.0
CABBAGE (RED)	0.0
CABBAGE (SAVOY)	0.0
CAKE & PASTRY FLOUR	0.6
CAROB FLOUR	0.0
CARROTS (FROZEN, COOKED)	0.0
CARROTS (RAW)	0.0
CATSUP	0.9
CAULIFLOWER	0.0
CELERY (PASCAL, RAW)	0.0
CHERRIES (SOUR, CANNED, WATER)	0.0
CHICKEN BREAST (ROASTED)	0.5
CHICKEN CHOW MEIN	0.0
CHICKEN DRUMSTICK (NO SKIN, ROASTED)	0.8
CHICKEN LIVER	0.9
CLAMS	0.4
COLLARDS	0.0
CORN FLAKES	0.0
CORN GRITS (WHITE)	0.0
CORN GRITS (YELLOW)	0.0
COTTAGE CHEESE (LOWFAT 2%)	0.6
COTTAGE CHEESE (UNCREAMED)	0.2
CRABMEAT	0.6
CRANBERRY SAUCE (SWEATENED, CANNED)	0.0
CREAM OF WHEAT	0.0

EGGPLANT	**0.0**
EGGS (WHITE, RAW)	**0.0**
ENDIVE	**0.0**
ENGLISH MUFFINS (PLAIN)	**0.9**
EVAPORATED MILK (SKIM)	**0.2**
FLOUNDER (BAKED, NO FAT)	**0.3**
FROSTED FLAKES CEREAL	**0.0**
FRUIT COCKTAIL (CANNED, HEAVY SYRUP)	**0.0**
FRUIT COCKTAIL (CANNED, JUICE)	**0.0**
GELATIN DESSERT	**0.0**
GRAPE JUICE (CANNED)	**0.0**
GRAPEFRUIT (CANNED, SYRUP)	**0.0**
GRAPEFRUIT (RAW)	**0.0**
GRAPEFRUIT JUICE (SWEETENED)	**0.0**
GRAPEFRUIT JUICE (UNSWEETENED)	**0.0**
GRAPE-NUTS CEREAL	**0.0**
GREAT NORTHERN BEANS (DRY, DRAINED)	**0.3**
HONEY	**1.0**
HONEYDEW MELON	**0.0**
ITALIAN BREAD	**0.5**
JERUSALEM-ARTICHOKE	**0.0**
KIWIFRUIT	**0.0**
KOHLRABI	**0.0**
LEMONS (RAW)	**0.0**
LENTILS	**0.3**
LETTUCE (BUTTER-HEAD)	**0.0**
LETTUCE (CRISP-HEAD)	**0.9**
LETTUCE (LOOSE LEAF)	**0.0**
LIMA BEANS	**0.3**

MACARONI	0.6
MALT-O-MEAL	1.0
MARSHMALLOWS	0.0
MELBA TOAST	0.0
MILK (NONFAT)	0.5
MUSHROOMS (CANNED)	0.0
MUSHROOMS (RAW)	0.0
MUSTARD GREENS	0.0
NONFAT DRY MILK	0.1
OKRA	0.0
ONION SOUP	0.0
ONIONS (RAW)	0.0
ONIONS (RAW, SPRING)	0.0
ORANGE & GRAPEFRUIT JUICE	0.0
ORANGE (RAW)	0.0
ORANGE JUICE (CANNED)	0.0
ORANGE JUICE (FRESH)	0.0
OYSTERS (RAW)	0.9
PAPAYA	0.0
PARSNIPS	0.0
PEA BEANS (DRY)	0.3
PEACHES (CANNED, HEAVY SYRUP)	0.0
PEACHES (CANNED, JUICE)	0.0
PEACHES (DRIED)	0.8
PEACHES (FRESH)	0.0
PEAR (CANNED, HEAVY SYRUP)	0.0
PEAR (CANNED, JUICE)	0.0
PEAS (CANNED, GREEN)	0.6
PEAS (FRESH, GREEN)	0.0
PEAS (POD)	0.0
PEPPERS (HOT GREEN CHILI)	0.0

PEPPERS (HOT RED CHILI)	0.0
PEPPERS (SWEET GREEN)	0.0
PEPPERS (SWEET RED)	0.0
PINEAPPLE (CANNED, HEAVY SYRUP)	0.0
PINEAPPLE (CANNED, JUICE)	0.0
PINEAPPLE JUICE (UNSWEETENED)	1.0
PINTO BEANS	0.3
PITA BREAD	0.8
PLANTAINS	0.0
PLUMS (CANNED, HEAVY SYRUP)	0.0
PLUMS (CANNED, JUICE)	0.0
PLUMS (FRESH)	0.0
POPCORN (AIR-POPPED)	0.0
POTATOES (BAKED, NO SKIN)	0.0
POTATOES (BAKED, WITH SKIN)	0.0
POTATOES (BOILED)	0.0
PRODUCT 19 CEREAL	0.0
PRUNE JUICE	0.0
PRUNES (DRIED)	0.0
PUMPKIN (FRESH)	0.0
RAISINS	0.9
RASPBERRIES (SWEETENED)	0.5
RED KIDNEY BEANS	0.3
REFRIED BEANS	0.8
RHUBARB (SWEETENED)	0.0
RICE (BROWN)	0.9
RICE (WHITE)	0.0
RICE KRISPIES CEREAL	0.0
SAUERKRAUT	0.0
SEAWEED (SPIRULINA)	0.6
SELF-RISING FLOUR (UNSIFTED)	0.4

SHRIMP	**0.2**
SNAP BEAN (GREEN)	**0.0**
SNAP BEAN (YELLOW)	**0.0**
SOLE (BAKED, NO FAT)	**0.3**
SOY SAUCE	**0.0**
SPAGHETTI (FIRM)	**0.6**
SPAGHETTI (SOFT)	**0.9**
SPECIAL K CEREAL	**1.0**
SPINACH (CANNED)	**0.8**
SPINACH (FRESH)	**0.0**
SPINACH (FROZEN)	**0.0**
SUPER SUGAR CRISP CEREAL	**1.0**
SWEET POTATOES (BAKED)	**0.0**
SWEETPOTATOES (CANNED)	**0.0**
SWEETPOTATOES (CANNED, MASHED)	**0.9**
SYRUP (LIGHT, CHOCOLATE FLAVORED)	**1.0**
TANGERINE JUICE	**1.0**
TANGERINES (CANNED, LIGHT SYRUP)	**0.0**
TANGERINES (FRESH)	**0.0**
TOMATO JUICE	**0.0**
TOMATO PUREE	**0.0**
TOMATOES (FRESH)	**0.0**
TRIX CEREAL	**1.0**
TUNA (CANNED, LIGHT, WATER)	**0.2**
TURKEY (LIGHT & DARK, ROASTED)	**0.8**
TURKEY (ROASTED)	**0.5**
TURKEY LOAF	**0.5**
TURNIP GREENS (FRESH)	**0.0**
TURNIP GREENS (FROZEN)	**0.9**
TURNIPS	**0.0**

VEGETABLE JUICE	0.0
VEGETABLES (MIXED)	0.0
WATER CHESTNUTS	0.0
WHEAT FLOUR (ALL-PURPOSE, SIFTED	0.4
WHEAT FLOUR (ALL-PURPOSE, UNSIFTED)	0.3
WHEATIES CEREAL	1.0
WHOLE-WHEAT FLOUR	0.6
YOGURT (FRUIT, NONFAT MILK)	0.9
YOGURT (NONFAT MILK)	0.0

FP 'YELLOW' TABLE

Eat foods from this table for 2 weeks along with foods from the FP 'Green' table.

Name of food	FP value
ALL-BRAN CEREAL	1.1
BAGELS (EGG)	1.3
BAGELS (PLAIN)	1.3
BAMBOO SHOOTS (CANNED)	2.3
BEANS (PORK, TOMATO SAUCE)	2.0
BEEF (LEAN & FAT, BOTTOM ROUND)	2.4
BEEF (LEAN, BOTTOM ROUND)	1.4
BEEF (LEAN, CHUCK BLADE)	2.1
BEEF BROTH (BOULLION)	1.5
BEEF GRAVY	2.5
BEEF LIVER	1.4
BEEF NOODLE SOUP	2.7
BEEF ROAST (LEAN, EYE O RND)	1.0
BEEF ROAST (LEAN & FAT, EYE O RND)	2.3
BEEF ROAST (LEAN, RIBS)	2.4
BEEF STEAK (LEAN, SIRLOIN, BROIL)	1.2
BOSTON BROWN BREAD	2.3
BREADCRUMBS	1.7
BROWN GRAVY (DRY MIX)	3.0
CANTALOUP	2.3
CHEERIOS CEREAL	2.3
CHESTNUTS (ROASTED)	2.7
CHICKEN (CANNED)	1.6
CHICKEN (LIGHT & DARK, STEWED)	1.1
CHICKEN BREAST (FRIED, BATTERED)	2.3

CHICKEN BREAST (FRIED, FLOUR)	1.4
CHICKEN DRUMSTICK, (FRIED, FLOUR)	2.4
CHICKEN GRAVY (DRY MIX)	3.0
CHICKEN NOODLE SOUP	2.3
CHICKEN RICE SOUP	2.3
CHICKEN ROLL	1.8
CHICKPEAS	1.3
CHOCOLATE MILK (LOWFAT 1%)	1.7
CHOCOLATE MILK (LOWFAT 2%)	2.8
CLAM CHOWDER (MANHATTAN)	2.3
COCOA POWDER (NO FAT DRY MILK)	1.5
CORN (CREAM, CANNED)	1.1
CORN (RAW, WHITE)	1.5
CORN (RAW, YELLOW)	2.3
CORNED BEEF (CANNED)	2.0
CORNMEAL	2.0
COTTAGE CHEESE (FRUIT)	1.7
COTTAGE CHEESE (LARGE CURDS, CREAMED)	1.6
CRACKED-WHEAT BREAD	2.3
CRACKED-WHEAT BREAD	1.7
DANDELION GREENS	2.3
DATES	1.1
DUCK (ROASTED)	2.3
EGG NOODLES	1.3
FIGS (DRIED)	1.5
FISH STICKS	2.3
FLOUNDER (BAKED IN BUTTER)	1.7
FLOUNDER (BAKED IN MARGARINE)	1.7
FRENCH BREAD	1.9
FROOT LOOPS CEREAL	2.3

GOLDEN GRAHAMS CEREAL	2.3
GREEN PEAS (SOUP)	1.5
HADDOCK (BREADED, FRIED)	2.4
HALIBUT (BROILED, BUTTER & LEMON JUICE)	1.4
HONEY NUT CHEERIOS CEREAL	1.5
ICE MILK (VANILLA, 3%)	2.8
KALE	1.1
LAMB (LEG, LEAN & FAT, ROASTED)	2.7
LAMB (LEG, LEAN, ROASTED)	1.4
LAMB CHOPS (ARM, LEAN, BRAISED)	2.0
LAMB CHOPS (LOIN, LEAN, BROIL)	1.4
LAMB RIB (LEAN, ROASTED)	2.1
LUCKY CHARMS CEREAL	1.5
MILK (1% LOW FAT)	1.1
MILK (2% LOW FAT)	2.5
MISO	2.1
MIXED GRAIN BREAD	1.7
MOZZARELLA CHESE (NONFAT MILK)	2.8
OATMEAL (FLAVORED)	1.8
OATMEAL (PLAIN)	2.3
OATMEAL BREAD	2.4
PIZZA (CHEESE)	2.9
POPCORN (SYRUP)	2.3
PORK (CURED, HAM, LEAN)	1.1
PORK (LUNCHEON MEAT, HAM, LEAN & FAT)	2.7
PORK (LUNCHEON MEAT, HAM, LEAN)	1.2
PORK (ROASTED HAM, LEAN)	1.8
PORK CHOP LOIN (BROILED, LEAN)	1.6
PORK CHOP LOIN (FRIED, LEAN)	2.8
PORK RIBS (ROASTED, LEAN)	2.3

PORK SHOULDER (BRAISED, LEAN)	1.6
PRETZELS	2.3
PUMPERNICKEL BREAD	1.8
PUMPKIN (CANNED)	1.5
RAISIN BRAN CEREAL	1.5
RAISIN BREAD	2.3
ROAST BEEF SANDWICH	2.7
ROLLS (FRANKFURTER & HAMBURGER)	3.0
ROLLS (HARD)	1.8
RYE BREAD (LIGHT)	2.0
SALMON (CANNED)	1.3
SALMON (RED, BAKED)	1.1
SALMON (SMOKED)	2.0
SARDINES (CANNED, OIL, ATLANTIC)	2.0
SCALLOPS (BREADED)	3.0
SHREDDED WHEAT CEREAL	1.5
SHRIMP (FRIED, NOT BREADED, NOT BATTERED)	2.8
SOLE (BAKED IN MARGARINE)	1.7
SOLE (BAKED IN BUTTER)	1.7
SOYBEANS	2.4
SPAGHETTI (TOMATO SAUCE, CHEESE)	1.5
SQUASH (SUMMER)	2.3
SQUASH (WINTER)	2.3
STEAK (BROILED, SIRLOIN)	2.9
SUGAR SMACKS CEREAL	2.3
TOFU	2.5
TOMATO PASTE	1.0
TOMATOES (CANNED)	2.3
TORTILLAS (CORN)	2.3
TOTAL CEREAL	1.5

TROUT (BROILED, BUTTER)	1.9
TUNA (CANNED, LIGHT, OIL, DRAINNED)	1.3
TUNA SALAD	2.6
TURKEY AND GRAVY	2.6
TURKEY HAM (CURED)	1.2
VEAL CUTLET (BROILED, ROASTED, BRAISED)	1.8
VEAL RIB (BROILED, ROASTED, BRAISED)	2.7
VEGETABLE & BEEF SOUP	1.5
VIENNA BREAD	2.3
WATERMELON	3.0
WHEAT BREAD	2.0
WHITE BREAD	2.2
WHITE BREAD CRUMBS	2.3
WHITE BREAD CUBES	2.3
WHOLE-WHEAT BREAD	2.1
YOGURT (PLAIN, LOW FAT MILK)	1.5

FP 'RED' TABLE

Avoid the foods in this table during this 2 week rotation.

Name of food	FP value
ALMONDS (SLIVERED)	11.7
AMERICAN CHEESE	8.1
AMERICAN CHEESE SPREAD	5.4
APPLE JUICE (CANNED)	4.5
APPLE PIE	22.5
APPLE PIE (FRIED)	31.5
APPLES (RAW, UNPEELED)	4.5
APPLESAUCE (CANNED, SWEETENED)	4.5
APPLESAUCE (CANNED,UNSWEETENED)	4.5
AVOCADOS (CALIFORNIA)	33.8
AVOCADOS (FLORIDA)	24.3
BANANAS	4.5
BARBECUE SAUCE	4.5
BEAN WITH BACON SOUP	3.4
BEANS (CANNED, FRANKFURTER)	4.3
BEANS (PORK, SWEET SAUCE)	3.4
BEEF (LEAN & FAT CHUCK BLADE)	5.3
BEEF AND VEGETABLE STEW	3.1
BEEF POTPIE	6.4
BEEF ROAST (LEAN & FAT, RIBS)	6.2
BISCUIT BAKING MIX	6.8
BLACKBERRIES (RAW)	4.5
BLUE CHEESE	6.0
BLUE CHEESE SALAD DRESSING	36.0
BLUEBERRIES (RAW)	4.5
BLUEBERRY MUFFINS	7.5
BLUEBERRY PIE	20.0

BOLOGNA	10.3
BOUILLON (DEHYDRATED)	4.5
BRAN MUFFINS	6.0
BRAUNSCHWEIGER	10.1
BRAZIL NUTS	21.4
BREAD STUFFING (DRY MIX)	15.5
BROWNIES WITH NUTS	27.0
BUTTER	414.0
CAMEMBERT CHEESE	5.1
CANDY (MILK CHOCOLATE, ALMONDS)	15.0
CANDY (MILK CHOCOLATE, PEANUTS)	12.4
CANDY (MILK CHOCOLATE, PLAIN)	20.3
CANDY (MILK CHOCOLATE, RICE CRISPIES)	15.8
CAP'N CRUNCH CEREAL	13.5
CARAMEL	13.5
CARROT CAKE (CREME CHESE FROSTING)	23.4
CASHEW NUTS (DRY ROASTD)	14.6
CASHEW NUTS (ROASTED, OIL)	13.5
CELERY SEED	4.5
CEREAL (100% NATURAL)	9.0
CHEDDAR CHEESE	5.8
CHEESE CRACKERS (PEANUT SANDWICH)	9.0
CHEESE CRACKERS (PLAIN)	4.5
CHEESE SAUCE WITH MILK	4.8
CHEESEBURGER	4.5
CHEESECAKE	17.1
CHERRIES (RAW, SWEET)	4.5
CHERRY PIE	19.3
CHERRY PIE (FRIED)	31.5
CHICKEN A LA KING	5.9
CHICKEN AND NOODLES	3.7

CHICKEN DRUMSTICK (FRIED, BATTERED)	3.3
CHICKEN FRANKFURTER	6.8
CHICKEN GRAVY (CANNED)	12.6
CHICKEN POTPIE	6.3
CHILI	3.8
CHOCOLATE (SWEET, DARK)	45.0
CHOCOLATE (FOR BAKING, BITTER)	22.5
CHOCOLATE CHIP COOKIES	20.3
CHOCOLATE MILK (REGULAR)	4.5
CHOCOLATE PUDDING	4.5
CHOCOLATE SHAKE	4.5
CHOP SUEY (BEEF & PORK)	3.1
CHOW MEIN NOODLES	8.3
CLAM CHOWDER (NEW ENGLAND, MILK)	3.5
CLUB SODA	4.5
COCOA POWDER (REGULAR)	4.5
COCONUT (RAW)	67.5
COCONUT (SHREDDED, DRIED, SWEETENED)	49.5
COFFEE	4.5
COFFEE CREAM (LIGHT)	34.5
COFFEECAKE (CRUMB)	6.8
COLA (DIET)	4.5
COLA (REGULAR)	4.5
CONDENSED MILK (SWEETENED)	5.1
CORN CHIPS	20.3
CORN MUFFINS	7.5
CORN OIL	981000.0
CRACKERS (SNACK)	4500.0
CRANBERRY JUICE COCKTAL	4.5
CREAM CHEESE	22.5

CREAM OF CHICKEN SOUP (MILK)	7.1
CREAM OF CHICKEN SOUP (WATER)	10.5
CREAM OF MUSHROM SOUP (MILK)	10.5
CREAM OF MUSHROOM SOUP (WATER)	20.3
CREME PIE	31.3
CROISSANTS	10.8
CUCUMBER (WITH PEEL)	4.5
CUSTARD (BAKED)	5.2
CUSTARD PIE	8.7
DANISH PASTRY (FRUIT)	14.6
DANISH PASTRY (PLAIN)	15.2
DEVIL'S FOOD CAKE (CHOCOLATE FROSTING)	13.6
DOUGHNUTS (CAKE TYPE, PLAIN)	18.0
DOUGHNUTS (YEAST-LEAVENED, GLAZED)	19.5
EGGS (FRIED)	5.3
EGGS (HARD-BOILED)	3.8
EGGS (POACHED)	3.8
EGGS (SCRAMBLED)	4.5
EGGS (WHOLE, RAW)	3.8
EGGS (YOLK, RAW)	7.5
ENCHILADA	3.6
ENG MUFFIN (BACON, EGG, CHEESE)	4.5
EVAPORATED MILK (WHOLE)	5.0
FETA CHEESE	6.8
FIG BARS	9.0
FILBERTS (HAZELNUTS)	21.6
FISH SANDWICH (CHEESE)	6.5
FISH SANDWICH (NO CHEESE)	6.8
FONDANT	4.5
FRANKFURTER	11.7

FRENCH SALAD DRESSING (LOW CAL)	9000.0
FRENCH SALAD DRESSING (REGULAR)	40500.0
FRENCH TOAST	5.3
FRUIT JELLIES	4.5
FRUIT PUNCH DRINK (CANNED)	4.5
FRUITCAKE	13.9
FUDGE, CHOCOLATE, PLAIN	9.5
GINGER ALE	4.5
GINGERBREAD CAKE	9.8
GRAHAM CRACKER (PLAIN)	4.5
GRAPE DRINK (CANNED)	4.5
GRAPE SODA	4.5
GRAPES (RAW)	4.5
GROUND BEEF (BROILED, LEAN & FAT)	4.1
GROUND BEEF (BROILED, LEAN)	3.4
GUM DROPS	4.5
HALF AND HALF (CREAM)	18.0
HARD CANDY	4.5
HERRING (PICKLED)	3.4
HOLLANDAISE (WATER)	18.0
ICE CREAM (VANLLA,11% FAT)	13.6
ICE CREAM (VANLLA,16% FAT)	25.9
ICE MILK (VANILLA, 4% FAT)	4.9
IMITATION CREAMER (POWDERED)	4500.0
IMITATION SOUR DRESSING	21.9
IMITATION WHIPPED TOPING	3600.0
ITALIAN SALAD DRESSING (LOW CAL)	4.5
ITALIAN SALAD DRESSING (REGULAR)	40500.0
JAMS AND FRUIT PRESERVES	4.5
JELLY BEANS	4.5
LAMB CHOPS (ARM, LEAN & FAT, BRAISED)	3.4

LAMB CHOPS (LOIN, LEAN & FAT, BROIL)	3.3
LAMB RIB (LEAN & FAT, ROASTED)	6.5
LARD	922500.0
LEMON JUICE	4.5
LEMON MERINGUE PIE	12.5
LEMONADE	4.5
LEMON-LIME SODA	4.5
LIMEADE	4.5
LIQUOR (GIN, RUM, VODKA, WHISKY, COGNAC...)	4.5
MACADAMIA NUTS (OIL ROASTED)	46.4
MACARONI AND CHEESE	5.8
MALTED MILK (CHOCOLATE)	4.5
MALTED MILK (REGULAR)	4.1
MANGO (RAW)	4.5
MARGARINE (REGULAR, HARD)	49500.0
MARGARINE (IMITATION 40% FAT)	396.0
MARGARINE (REGULAR, HARD, 80% FAT)	409.5
MARGARINE (REGULR, SOFT)	49500.0
MARGARINE (REGULR, SOFT, 80% FAT)	823.5
MARGARINE (SPREAD, HARD, 60% FAT)	310.5
MARGARINE (SPREAD, SOFT, 60% FAT)	621.0
MAYONNAISE (IMITATION)	13500.0
MAYONNAISE (REGULAR)	49500.0
MAYONNAISE SALAD DRESSING	22500.0
MILK (WHOLE)	4.5
MINESTRONE SOUP	3.4
MIXED NUTS (DRY ROASTED, NO HONEY)	16.9
MIXED NUTS (OIL ROASTED, NO HONEY)	14.4
MOLASSES	4.5
MOZZARELLA CHEESE (WHOLE MILK)	4.5

MUENSTER CHEESE	5.8
MUSHROOM GRAVY	9.0
MUSTARD (YELLOW)	4.5
NATURE VALLEY GRANOLA CEREAL	7.5
NECTARINES	4.5
OATMEAL & RAISIN COOKIES	15.0
OCEAN PERCH (FRIED, BREADED)	3.1
OLIVE OIL	972000.0
OLIVES (BLACK)	9000.0
OLIVES (GREEN)	9000.0
ONION RINGS	22.5
ORANGE SODA	4.5
OYSTERS (FRIED, BREADED)	4.5
PANCAKES (BUCKWHEAT)	4.5
PANCAKES (PLAIN)	4.5
PARMESAN CHEESE	3.7
PEACH PIE	18.9
PEANUT BUTTER	7.2
PEANUT BUTTER COOKIE	15.8
PEANUT OIL	972000.0
PEANUTS (OIL-ROASTED)	7.9
PEAR (FRESH)	4.5
PECAN PIE	4.5
PECANS (HALVES)	41.1
PICKLES (CUCUMBER)	4.5
PICKLES (CUCUMBER, DILL)	4.5
PICKLES (CUCUMBER, SWEET)	4.5
PIE CRUST	20.9
PINE NUTS	38.3
PINEAPPLE (FRESH)	4.5
PINEAPPLE-GRAPEFRUIT JUICE DRINK	4.5

PISTACHIO NUTS	10.5
POPCORN (VEGETABLE OIL)	13.5
POPSICLE	4.5
PORK (CURED, BACON)	6.8
PORK (CURED, HAM, LEAN & FAT)	3.7
PORK (LINK)	6.0
PORK (LUNCHEON MEAT, CANNED)	11.7
PORK CHOP LOIN (BROILED, LEAN & FAT)	3.7
PORK CHOP LOIN (FRIED, LEAN & FAT)	5.8
PORK FRESH (ROASTED HAM, LEAN & FAT)	4.1
PORK RIBS (ROASTED, LEAN & FAT)	4.3
PORK SHOULDER (BRAISED, LEAN & FAT)	4.3
POTATO CHIPS	31.5
POTATO SALAD (MAYONNAISE)	13.5
POTATOES (AU GRATIN)	9.0
POTATOES (FRENCH FRIES, BAKED)	9.0
POTATOES (FRENCH FRIES, FRIED)	18.0
POTATOES (HASHED BROWN)	16.2
POTATOES (MASHED)	13.5
POTATOES (SCALLOPED)	9.9
POUND CAKE	16.3
PROVOLONE CHEESE	5.1
PUMPKIN AND SQUASH KERNELS	8.4
PUMPKIN PIE	13.1
QUICHE LORRAINE	16.6
RADISHES	4.5
RELISH (SWEET)	4.5
RICE PUDDING	4.5
RICOTTA CHEESE (SKIM MILK)	3.1
RICOTTA CHEESE (WHOLE MILK)	5.1
ROLLS (DINNER)	9.0

ROLLS (HOAGIE OR SUBMARINE)	3.3
ROOT BEER	4.5
RYE WAFERS (WHOLE-GRAIN)	4.5
SAFFLOWER OIL	981000.0
SALAMI (DRY)	6.3
SALAMI (NOT DRY)	6.2
SALTINES	4.5
SANDWICH SPREAD (BEEF & PORK)	13.5
SAUSAGE (BROWN AND SERVE)	11.3
SEAWEED (KELP)	4.5
SEMI SWEET CHOCOLATE	39.2
SESAME SEEDS	9.0
SHEETCAKE (NO FROSTING)	14.7
SHEETCAKE (WHITE FROSTING)	21.0
SHERBET	8.2
SHORTBREAD COOKIE	4.5
SNACK CAKES (DEVIL'S FOOD & CRÈME)	18.0
SNACK CAKES (SPONGE & CRÈME)	22.5
SOUR CREAM	30.9
SOYBEAN OIL (HYDROGENATED)	981000.0
SOYBEAN-COTTONSEED OIL (HYDROGENATED)	981000.0
SPAGHETTI (MEATBALLS, TOMATO SAUCE)	3.8
SPINACH SOUFFLE	7.4
STRAWBERRIES (FRESH)	4.5
STRAWBERRIES (FROZEN, SWEETENED)	4.5
SUGAR (BROWN)	4.5
SUGAR (WHITE)	4.5
SUGAR COOKIE	27.0
SUNFLOWER OIL	981000.0
SUNFLOWER SEEDS	10.5

SWEET POTATOE PIE	13500.0
SWISS CHEESE	4.5
SWISS CHEESE	4.5
SYRUP (CORN, MAPLE)	4.5
SYRUP (THICK, CHOCOLATE FLAVORED)	11.3
TACO	5.5
TAHINI	12.0
TAPIOCA PUDDING	7.5
TARTAR SAUCE	36000.0
TEA (INSTANT, SWEETENED)	4.5
THOUSAND ISLAND DRESSING	27000.0
TOASTER PASTRIES	13.5
TOMATO & VEGETABLE SOUP	4.5
TOMATO SOUP (MILK)	4.5
TOMATO SOUP (WATER)	4.5
TURKEY PATTIES (BATTERED, FRIED)	6.0
VANILLA PUDDING	22.5
VANILLA SHAKE	3.7
VANILLA WAFERS	15.8
VEGETARIAN SOUP	4.5
VIENNA SAUSAGE	9.0
VINEGAR (CIDER)	4.5
VINEGAR AND OIL SALAD DRESSING	36000.0
WAFFLES	5.1
WALNUTS (BLACK)	10.3
WALNUTS (ENGLISH)	19.6
WHEAT CRACKERS	4.5
WHIPPED TOPPING	29.3
WHIPPING CREAM (HEAVY)	79.2
WHIPPING CREAM (LIGHT)	66.6
WHITE CAKE (WHITE FROSTING)	15.5

WHITE SAUCE (MILK)	5.9
WHOLE-WHEAT WAFERS	9.0
YELLOW CAKE (CHOCOLATE FROSTING)	12.8
YOGURT (WHOLE MILK)	3.9
EGG NOG	9.5
PARMESAN CHEESE	3.2

The Plateau-proof Diet Cardio – A healthier heart version of the Plateau-proof Diet

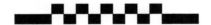

The plateau-proof diet cardio makes a distinction between total fat and saturated fat in the diet whereas the plateau-proof diet doesn't. Saturated fats may increase your risk for cardiovascular disease when consumed excessively. Since it eliminates foods with high saturated fat content, the plateau-proof diet cardio is a healthier version of the plateau-proof diet. I recommend the plateau-proof diet cardio over the plateau-proof diet because it may affect a more rapid weight loss and a healthier cardiovascular profile.

The plateau-proof diet cardio formulas

Like the plateau-proof diet, the plateau-proof cardio diet uses the CP and FP formulas. The plateau-proof diet however includes a saturated fat index in its formulas, which is not used in the plateau-proof diet formulas.

The CP and FP formulas for the plateau-proof cardio diets are:

$$CP = [(2 \times grams\ of\ carbs \times fiber\ index)\ /\ grams\ of\ protein] + SFi$$

SFi is the saturated fat index.

$$FP = [(4.5 \times grams\ of\ fats)\ /\ grams\ of\ protein] + SFi$$

Derivation of the saturated fat index

The saturated fat index is designed to eliminate foods that contribute more than 20% of their total fat as saturated fat.

The first step in the derivation of the saturated fat index divides total fat by unsaturated fat (total fat / unsaturated fat).

A hundredth of a point (0.01) is added to CP and FP for every hundredth (0.01) increase in (total fat / unsaturated fat) between 1 and 1.24. When (total fat / unsaturated fat) = 1.25, 20% of fats are saturated.

When (total fat / unsaturated fat) values are greater than or equal to 1.25, a tenth of a point (0.1) is added to CP and FP for every hundredth point (0.01) increase in the value of (total fat / unsaturated fat).

How to use the plateau-proof diet cardio

The instructions for using the plateau-proof diet cardio are the same as those for the plateau-proof diet discussed in the previous chapter:

1) Start the diet with the CP 'Green' and 'Yellow' Tables. Make balanced meals out of the food items in these tables. Eat as wide a variety of foods as you are able to. Do this for 4

weeks. Avoid items in the 'Red' table. *[Note: if you are just getting off a low-carb diet program (within 2 weeks), start the plateau-proof diet with FP 'Green' and 'Yellow' tables.]*

2) At the end of 4 weeks, eat foods from the FP 'Green' and 'Yellow' tables for 2 weeks. Eat the widest variety of foods possible. Avoid foods in the 'Red' table. You probably are going to be at the peak of your weight loss from the CP rotation when you start the FP rotation. Once you are in the FP rotation, your rate of weight loss may be significantly lower than it was on the CP rotation. You should however complete this 2 week rotation before going back to the CP rotation. Remember that this is the strategy for avoiding the dreaded weight loss plateau. *Always try to balance your meals, and avoid eating the same items repeatedly.*

3) At the end of two weeks, go back to the CP rotation and keep alternating until you achieve complete weight loss. *Keep a daily record of the food items you eat and your weight.* When you achieve your desired weight loss, continue the diet with fewer restrictions to maintain your new lean body.

How much food should you eat?

There are many factors that determine how much food is required by your body each day. These factors include lean body mass and level of activity. Since no two people are identical in this regard, it is impractical to assign a fixed quantity of food for everyone. A more practical approach for the plateau-proof diet cardio is that you start the diet by cutting down your normal portion modestly. It would be beneficial to start by cutting down about 10 – 20 % of your original portion in the first rotation (4 weeks). You should then cut down an additional 5 – 10 % during each subsequent rotation. The minimum daily amount of food that you should eat after cutting down the portion size should be approximately 400 grams (14.1 ounces). You may not experience a robust weight loss until your daily food intake approaches the recommended daily minimum; however, your cardiovascular risk factors should improve from the beginning. When it comes to portion size, it is more important to start slowly and finish strongly, than to start strongly and never finish. In other words, it may be more beneficial to set your mentality for a marathon rather than a sprint.

If you believe that the cause of your weight problem is overeating and you are unable to sustain a portion restricting diet, please seek immediate help from your health care provider.

When should you eat?

It doesn't matter when you eat. You can eat at any time. Some studies have suggested that people who eat breakfast tend to lose weight better than people who don't eat breakfast. Also, it is better to eat your meals in many small portions throughout the day as opposed to one large portion.

The plateau-proof diet cardio and prepackaged foods

You can evaluate prepackaged foods on an individual bases for compliance with the plateau-proof diet cardio guidelines. Avoid prepackaged foods that contain trans fats and those that are high in sodium (salt).

1) Evaluating a food for the CP rotation
To evaluate a prepackaged food for the CP rotation, read its nutrition label and enter the amount of protein, carbohydrate, and fiber into the CP formula:

$$CP = [(2 \text{ x grams of carbs x fiber index}) / \text{ grams of protein}] + SFi$$

Convert grams of fiber into the fiber index using the table below:

Fiber content	Fiber index
- Very high-fiber (≥ 10 g per serving)	= 0.25
- High-fiber (≥ 5 g per serving)	= 0.50
- Moderate fiber(≥ 1 g per serving)	= 0.75
- Low or no fiber (< 1 g per serving)	= 1.00

Add the saturated fat index (SFi).

If the CP value is equal to or less than 2.0, the prepackaged food is a CP 'Green' table food. If the CP value is equal to or less than 10.0 but greater than 2.0, the prepackaged food belongs in the

CP 'Yellow' table. In either case, this food can be eaten during the 4 week CP rotation. If the CP value is greater than 10.0, the food cannot be eaten during the 4 week CP rotation.

2) *Evaluating a food for the FP rotation*

To evaluate a prepackaged food for the FP rotation, read its nutrition label, enter the amount of protein and total fat into the FP formula and add the SFi:

$$FP = [(4.5 \times grams\ of\ fats)\ /\ grams\ of\ protein] + SFi$$

If the FP value is equal to or less than 1.0, the food belongs in the FP 'Green' table and can be eaten during the 2 week FP rotation. If the FP value is equal to or less than 3.0 but greater than 1.0, the food belongs in the FP 'Yellow' table and can be eaten during the 2 week FP rotation. If the food has an FP value greater than 3.0, it cannot be eaten during the 2 week FP rotation.

Please note:

If a prepackaged food contains trans fats it should be avoided regardless of its CP or FP values.

CP 'GREEN' TABLE

Eat foods from this table for 4 weeks along with foods from the CP 'Yellow' table.

Name of food	CP value
ALFALFA SEEDS (SPROUTED, RAW)	1.5
ALMONDS (SLIVERED)	1.6
ASPARAGUS (CANNED)	3.0
ASPARAGUS (FROZEN)	1.5
BAMBOO SHOOTS (CANNED)	3.0
BEAN SPROUTS	2.5
BEEF (DRIED)	2.5
BEEF (LEAN, BOTTOM ROUND)	2.7
BEEF BROTH (BOULLION)	0.0
BEEF HEART (BRAISED)	0.0
BEEF LIVER (FRIED IN VEG OIL)	3.3
BEEF ROAST (LEAN, EYE O RND)	0.2
BLACK BEANS (COOKED, DRAINED)	1.4
BLACK-EYED PEAS, DRY, COOKED	1.5
BLUE CHEESE SALAD DRESSING	2.1
BOUILLON (DEHYDRATED)	2.0
BRAZIL NUTS	1.7
BROCCOLI (FROZEN, COOKED, DRAINED)	1.7
BROCCOLI (RAW, COOKED, DRAINED)	2.3
BRUSSELS SPROUTS	3.3
CABBAGE (CHINESE)	1.5
CELERY (PASCAL, RAW)	2.0
CHICKEN (CANNED)	0.2
CHICKEN (LIGHT & DARK, STEWED)	0.2
CHICKEN BREAST (FRIED VEG OIL, FLOUR)	0.3

CHICKEN BREAST (ROASTED)	0.0
CHICKEN DRUMSTICK (FRIED VEG OIL, BATTERED)	3.0
CHICKEN DRUMSTICK (ROASTED)	0.0
CHICKEN DRUMSTICK, (FRIED VEG OIL, FLOUR)	0.3
CHICKEN FRANKFURTER	1.2
CHICKEN LIVER	0.0
CHICKEN ROLL	0.2
CHICKPEAS	3.2
CHOP SUEY (BEEF & PORK)	3.4
CLAMS	0.4
CLUB SODA	2.0
COFFEE	2.0
COLA (DIET)	2.0
CORN OIL	2.1
COTTAGE CHEESE (UNCREAMED)	0.2
CRABMEAT	0.1
EGGS (FRIED IN VEG OIL)	0.5
EGGS (HARD-BOILED)	0.5
EGGS (POACHED)	0.4
EGGS (SCRAMBLED)	0.5
EGGS (WHITE, RAW)	0.0
EGGS (WHOLE, RAW)	0.5
EGGS (YOLK, RAW)	0.1
EVAPORATED MILK (NONFAT)	3.1
FILBERTS (HAZELNUTS)	2.5
FISH STICKS	1.3
FLOUNDER (BAKED IN VEG OIL)	0.0
FLOUNDER (BAKED, NO FAT)	0.0
GREAT NORTHERN BEANS (DRY, DRAINED)	2.9

HADDOCK (BREADED, FRIED IN VEG OIL)	1.0
HERRING (PICKLED)	3.4
LAMB (LEG, LEAN, ROASTED)	3.0
LENTILS	1.2
LIMA BEANS	3.1
LIQUOR (GIN, RUM, VODKA, WHISKY, COGNAC...)	2.0
MARGARINE (IMITATION 40% FAT)	2.2
MILK (NONFAT)	2.7
MIXED NUTS (DRY ROASTED, NO HONEY)	2.7
MIXED NUTS (OIL ROASTED, NO HONEY)	1.9
MUSTARD (YELLOW)	2.0
MUSTARD GREENS	2.0
NONFAT DRY MILK	3.0
OCEAN PERCH (FRIED IN VEG OIL, BREADED)	1.0
OLIVE OIL	2.2
OLIVES (BLACK)	2.0
OLIVES (GREEN)	2.0
OYSTERS (FRIED VEG OIL, BREADED)	2.1
OYSTERS (RAW)	0.9
PEANUT BUTTER	1.3
PEANUT OIL	2.2
PEANUTS (VEG OIL-ROASTED)	1.3
PEAS (POD)	3.3
PISTACHIO NUTS	1.8
PORK (CURED, HAM, LEAN)	0.1
PORK (LINK)	0.1
PORK (LUNCHEON MEAT, HAM, LEAN)	0.2
PORK (ROASTED HAM, LEAN)	2.7
PORK CHOP LOIN (BROILED, LEAN)	2.5

PORK CHOP LOIN (FRIED VEG OIL, LEAN)	3.3
PORK RIBS (ROASTED, LEAN)	3.2
PORK SHOULDER (BRAISED, LEAN)	2.9
PUMPKIN AND SQUASH KERNELS	1.6
RED KIDNEY BEANS	2.8
SAFFLOWER OIL	2.1
SALAMI (DRY)	2.9
SALMON (CANNED)	0.0
SALMON (RED, BAKED)	0.0
SALMON (SMOKED)	2.5
SARDINES (CANNED, VEG OIL, ATLANTIC)	0.1
SCALLOPS (BREADED)	1.5
SEAWEED (SPIRULINA)	0.9
SESAME SEEDS	1.0
SHRIMP	0.1
SHRIMP (FRIED VEG OIL, NOT BREADED / BATTERED)	1.6
SOLE (BAKED IN VEG OIL)	0.0
SOLE (BAKED, NO FAT)	0.0
SOY SAUCE	2.0
SOYBEAN OIL	2.2
SOYBEAN-COTTONSEED OIL	2.2
SOYBEANS	1.5
SPINACH (CANNED)	1.8
SPINACH (FRESH)	1.5
SPINACH (FROZEN)	2.5
SUNFLOWER OIL	2.1
SUNFLOWER SEEDS	1.7
TAHINI	2.0
TEA (BREWED, UNSWEETENED)	2.0
TOFU	0.7

TUNA (CANNED, LIGHT, OIL, DRAINNED)	0.1
TUNA (CANNED, LIGHT, WATER)	0.0
TUNA SALAD	1.3
TURKEY (LIGHT & DARK, ROASTED)	0.2
TURKEY (ROASTED)	0.0
TURKEY AND GRAVY	2.1
TURKEY HAM (CURED)	0.0
TURKEY LOAF	0.0
TURNIP GREENS (FROZEN)	3.2
VEGETABLE & BEEF SOUP	2.5
VINEGAR AND OIL SALAD DRESSING	2.1
WALNUTS (BLACK)	0.6
WALNUTS (ENGLISH)	2.0
YOGURT (NONFAT MILK)	2.8
BEET GREENS	3.0

CP 'YELLOW' TABLE

Eat foods from this table for 4 weeks along with foods from the CP 'Green' table.

Name of food	CP value
ALL-BRAN CEREAL	5.3
AMERICAN CHEESE SPREAD	9.6
ARTICHOKES (GLOBE, COOKED)	6.0
AVOCADOS (CALIFORNIA)	6.1
BEANS (CANNED, FRANKFURTER)	7.2
BEANS (PORK, SWEET SAUCE)	7.2
BEANS (PORK, TOMATO SAUCE)	5.5
BEEF (LEAN, CHUCK BLADE)	4.8
BEEF (REGULAR CHUCK BLADE)	6.0
BEEF (REGULAR, BOTTOM ROUND)	4.1
BEEF AND VEGETABLE STEW	5.9
BEEF GRAVY	7.6
BEEF NOODLE SOUP	3.6
BEEF POTPIE	6.7
BEEF ROAST (LEAN, RIBS)	4.1
BEEF ROAST (REGULAR, EYE O RND)	4.8
BEEF ROAST (REGULAR, RIBS)	6.0
BEEF STEAK (LEAN, SIRLOIN, BROIL)	3.6
BROWN GRAVY (DRY MIX)	9.3
CABBAGE (RED)	6.0
CABBAGE (SAVOY)	6.0
CARROTS (FROZEN, COOKED)	9.0
CASHEW NUTS (DRY ROASTD)	4.6
CASHEW NUTS (ROASTED, OIL)	3.7
CAULIFLOWER	4.5

CHICKEN A LA KING	6.3
CHICKEN AND NOODLES	5.3
CHICKEN BREAST (FRIED VEG OIL, BATTERED)	3.5
CHICKEN CHOW MEIN	5.1
CHICKEN GRAVY (CANNED)	5.4
CHICKEN GRAVY (DRY MIX)	9.3
CHICKEN NOODLE SOUP	4.5
CHICKEN POTPIE	8.1
CHICKEN RICE SOUP	3.5
CHILI	6.7
CHOCOLATE MILK (LOWFAT 1%)	6.7
CHOW MEIN NOODLES	8.8
CLAM CHOWDER (MANHATTAN)	6.0
CLAM CHOWDER (NEW ENGLAND, LOW-FAT MILK)	7.8
COLLARDS	3.8
CORN (RAW, WHITE)	9.5
CORNED BEEF (CANNED)	4.7
COTTAGE CHEESE (LOWFAT 2%)	8.7
CREAM OF CHICKEN SOUP (LOW-FAT MILK)	9.2
CREAM OF CHICKEN SOUP (WATER)	6.2
CREAM OF MUSHROM SOUP (LF MILK)	9.1
CREAM OF MUSHROOM SOUP (WATER)	9.2
DANDELION GREENS	5.3
DUCK (ROASTED)	4.9
ENCHILADA	9.6
ENDIVE	4.0
ENG MUFFIN (EGG, LOW-FAT CHEESE)	9.8
FISH SANDWICH (LOW-FAT CHEESE)	7.9

FISH SANDWICH (NO CHEESE)	7.0
FLOUNDER (BAKED IN VEG OIL)	5.8
FRANKFURTER	4.5
FRENCH TOAST	5.8
GREEN PEAS (SOUP)	4.7
GROUND BEEF (BROILED, LEAN)	4.8
GROUND BEEF (BROILED, REGULAR)	4.9
HALIBUT (BROILED, VEG OIL & LEMON JUICE)	6.2
KALE	3.5
KOHLRABI	7.3
LAMB (LEG, REGULAR, ROASTED)	5.5
LAMB CHOPS (ARM, LEAN, BRAISED)	3.7
LAMB CHOPS (ARM, REGULAR, BRAISED)	6.5
LAMB CHOPS (LOIN, LEAN, BROIL)	3.6
LAMB CHOPS (LOIN, REGULAR, BROIL)	6.5
LAMB RIB (LEAN, ROASTED)	4.6
LAMB RIB (REGULAR, ROASTED)	7.4
LETTUCE (BUTTER-HEAD)	4.0
LETTUCE (CRISP-HEAD)	4.4
LETTUCE (LOOSE LEAF)	4.0
MACADAMIA NUTS (OIL ROASTED)	3.6
MARGARINE (SPREAD, HARD, 60% FAT)	4.8
MARGARINE (SPREAD, SOFT, 60% FAT)	4.6
MELBA TOAST	8.0
MILK (1% LOW FAT)	6.3
MILK (2% LOW FAT)	8.8
MINESTRONE SOUP	5.5
MISO	4.7
MIXED GRAIN BREAD	9.6
MOZZARELLA CHEESE (LOW-FAT MILK)	8.5

MOZZARELLA CHESE (NONFAT MILK)	7.5
MUENSTER CHEESE	9.6
MUSHROOM GRAVY	8.7
MUSHROOMS (CANNED)	5.3
MUSHROOMS (RAW)	6.0
OATMEAL (PLAIN)	9.0
OKRA	4.5
ONION SOUP	8.0
ONIONS (RAW, SPRING)	4.0
PARMESAN CHEESE	9.8
PEA BEANS (DRY)	4.0
PEAS (CANNED, GREEN)	5.3
PEAS (FRESH, GREEN)	4.4
PECANS (HALVES)	5.1
PEPPERS (HOT GREEN CHILI)	8.0
PEPPERS (HOT RED CHILI)	8.0
PEPPERS (SWEET GREEN)	8.0
PEPPERS (SWEET RED)	8.0
PINE NUTS	5.1
PINTO BEANS	4.9
POPCORN (AIR-POPPED)	9.0
POPCORN (VEGETABLE OIL)	9.0
PORK (CURED, HAM, REGULAR)	4.1
PORK (LUNCHEON MEAT, CANNED)	4.1
PORK CHOP LOIN (BROILED, REGULAR)	4.6
PORK CHOP LOIN (FRIED, REGULAR)	4.8
PORK FRESH (ROASTED HAM, REGULAR)	4.3
PORK RIBS (ROASTED, REGULAR)	4.5
PORK SHOULDER (BRAISED, REGULAR)	4.6
PROVOLONE CHEESE	9.3
REFRIED BEANS	4.3

ROAST BEEF SANDWICH	5.5
RYE BREAD (LIGHT)	8.8
SALAMI (NOT DRY)	5.2
SANDWICH SPREAD (BEEF & PORK)	4.0
SAUERKRAUT	7.5
SNAP BEAN (GREEN)	4.5
SNAP BEAN (YELLOW)	4.5
SOLE (BAKED IN BUTTER)	5.8
SPAGHETTI (FIRM)	8.4
SPAGHETTI (MEATBALLS, TOMATO SAUCE)	5.0
SPINACH SOUFFLE	5.6
SQUASH (SUMMER)	8.0
STEAK (BROILED, SIRLOIN)	5.6
TACO	7.2
TOMATOES (FRESH)	7.5
TORTILLAS (CORN)	9.8
TROUT (BROILED, VEG OIL)	5.3
TURKEY PATTIES (BATTERED, FRIED)	4.2
TURNIP GREENS (FRESH)	6.0
VEAL CUTLET (BROILED, ROASTED, BRAISED)	5.3
VEAL RIB (BROILED, ROASTED, BRAISED)	5.6
VEGETABLE JUICE	8.3
VEGETABLES (MIXED)	5.6
VEGETARIAN SOUP	9.0
WHOLE-WHEAT FLOUR	8.0
WHOLE-WHEAT WAFERS	7.5
YOGURT (PLAIN, LOW FAT MILK)	7.5

CP 'RED' TABLE

Avoid the foods in this table during this 4 week rotation

Name of food	CP value
AMERICAN CHEESE	10.5
ANGELFOOD CAKE	18.0
APPLE JUICE (CANNED)	58000.0
APPLE PIE	37.7
APPLE PIE (FRIED)	36.2
APPLES (RAW, UNPEELED)	480.0
APPLES (DRIED, SULFURED)	630.0
APPLESAUCE (CANNED, SWEETENED)	1020.0
APPLESAUCE (CANNED,UNSWEETENED)	560.0
APRICOT (CANNED, HEAVY SYRUP)	110.0
APRICOT NECTAR	72.0
APRICOTS (CANNED, IN JUICE)	31.0
APRICOTS (DRIED)	27.5
APRICOTS (RAW)	18.0
AVOCADOS (FLORIDA)	11.0
BAGELS (EGG)	10.9
BAGELS (PLAIN)	10.9
BANANAS	54.0
BARBECUE SAUCE	4000.0
BARLEY (PEARLED, LIGHT)	14.8
BEER (LIGHT)	10.0
BEER (REGULAR)	26.0
BEETS (CANNED)	12.0
BEETS (COOKED, DRAINED)	14.0
BISCUIT BAKING MIX	14.0
BLACKBERRIES (RAW)	27.0
BLUE CHEESE	11.9

BLUEBERRIES (FROZEN, SWEETENED)	100.0
BLUEBERRIES (RAW)	40.0
BLUEBERRY MUFFINS	13.4
BLUEBERRY PIE	31.9
BOSTON BROWN BREAD	21.0
BRAN FLAKES (40%)	11.0
BRAN MUFFINS	12.1
BREAD STUFFING (DRY MIX)	11.3
BREADCRUMBS	11.3
BROWNIES WITH NUTS	22.1
BUCKWHEAT FLOUR (LIGHT, SIFTED)	19.5
BULGUR	13.7
BUTTER	15.6
BUTTERMILK (DRIED)	11.8
CABBAGE (COMMON)	10.5
CAKE & PASTRY FLOUR	21.7
CAMEMBERT CHEESE	11.4
CANDY (MILK CHOCOLATE, ALMONDS)	16.1
CANDY (MILK CHOCOLATE, PEANUTS)	10.6
CANDY (MILK CHOCOLATE, PLAIN)	25.6
CANDY (MILK CHOCOLATE, RICE CRISPIES)	27.4
CANTALOUP	22.0
CAP'N CRUNCH CEREAL	49.0
CARAMEL	50.7
CAROB FLOUR	42.0
CARROT CAKE (CREME CHESE FROSTING)	27.1
CARROTS (RAW)	12.0
CATSUP	27.6
CELERY SEED	10.0
CEREAL (100% NATURAL)	16.7

CHEDDAR CHEESE	12.5
CHEERIOS CEREAL	10.0
CHEESE CRACKERS (PEANUT SANDWICH)	10.0
CHEESE CRACKERS (PLAIN)	12.0
CHEESE SAUCE WITH MILK	12.4
CHEESEBURGER	10.9
CHEESECAKE	23.9
CHERRIES (RAW, SWEET)	22.0
CHERRIES (SOUR, CANNED, WATER)	44.0
CHERRY PIE	32.4
CHERRY PIE (FRIED)	37.2
CHESTNUTS (ROASTED)	30.4
CHOCOLATE (SWEET, DARK)	41.6
CHOCOLATE (FOR BAKING, BITTER)	16.7
CHOCOLATE CHIP COOKIES	30.7
CHOCOLATE MILK (LOWFAT 2%)	13.7
CHOCOLATE MILK (REGULAR)	17.7
CHOCOLATE PUDDING	18.3
CHOCOLATE SHAKE	24.0
COCOA POWDER (NO FAT DRY MILK)	14.7
COCOA POWDER (REGULAR)	16.3
COCONUT (RAW)	58.2
COCONUT (SHREDDED, DRIED, SWEETENED)	82.2
COFFEE CREAM (LIGHT)	18.3
COFFEECAKE (CRUMB)	20.3
COLA (REGULAR)	82000.0
CONDENSED MILK (SWEETENED)	27.9
CORN (CREAM, CANNED)	23.0
CORN (RAW, YELLOW)	14.3
CORN CHIPS	16.0

CORN FLAKES	24.0
CORN GRITS (WHITE)	20.7
CORN GRITS (YELLOW)	20.7
CORN MUFFINS	14.1
CORNMEAL	16.4
COTTAGE CHEESE (FRUIT)	12.4
COTTAGE CHEESE (LARGE CURDS, CREAMED)	12.1
CRACKED-WHEAT BREAD	12.0
CRACKED-WHEAT BREAD	11.0
CRACKERS (SNACK)	40.0
CRANBERRY JUICE COCKTAL	76000.0
CRANBERRY SAUCE (SWEATENED, CANNED)	216.0
CREAM CHEESE	11.8
CREAM OF WHEAT	14.0
CREME PIE	53.0
CROISSANTS	13.4
CUCUMBER (WITH PEEL)	200.0
CUSTARD (BAKED)	10.8
CUSTARD PIE	13.0
DANISH PASTRY (FRUIT)	16.9
DANISH PASTRY (PLAIN)	18.6
DATES	32.8
DEVIL'S FOOD CAKE (CHOCOLATE FROSTING)	35.4
DOUGHNUTS (CAKE TYPE, PLAIN)	16.2
DOUGHNUTS (YEAST-LEAVENED, GLAZED)	22.1
EGG NOG	19.4
EGG NOODLES	10.6
EGGPLANT	12.0

ENGLISH MUFFINS (PLAIN)	10.8
EVAPORATED MILK (WHOLE)	15.5
FETA CHEESE	11.9
FIG BARS	31.5
FIGS (DRIED)	20.3
FRENCH BREAD	10.9
FRENCH SALAD DRESSING (LOW CAL)	4000.0
FRENCH SALAD DRESSING (REGULAR)	2000.0
FROOT LOOPS CEREAL	25.0
FROSTED FLAKES CEREAL	52.0
FRUIT COCKTAIL (CANNED, HEAVY SYRUP)	96.0
FRUIT COCKTAIL (CANNED, JUICE)	58.0
FRUIT JELLIES	20000.0
FRUIT PUNCH DRINK (CANNED)	44000.0
FRUITCAKE	23.8
FUDGE, CHOCOLATE, PLAIN	53.0
GELATIN DESSERT	17.0
GINGER ALE	64000.0
GINGERBREAD CAKE	35.1
GOLDEN GRAHAMS CEREAL	24.0
GRAHAM CRACKER (PLAIN)	22.0
GRAPE DRINK (CANNED)	52000.0
GRAPE JUICE (CANNED)	76.0
GRAPE SODA	92000.0
GRAPEFRUIT (CANNED, SYRUP)	78.0
GRAPEFRUIT (RAW)	20.0
GRAPEFRUIT JUICE (SWEETENED)	56.0
GRAPEFRUIT JUICE (UNSWEETENED)	48.0
GRAPE-NUTS CEREAL	15.3
GRAPES (RAW)	1800.0

GUM DROPS	50000.0
HALF AND HALF (CREAM)	16.8
HARD CANDY	56000.0
HOLLANDAISE (WATER)	16.9
HONEY	558.0
HONEY NUT CHEERIOS CEREAL	15.3
HONEYDEW MELON	24.0
ICE CREAM (VANLLA,11% FAT)	29.1
ICE CREAM (VANLLA,16% FAT)	31.6
ICE MILK (VANILLA, 3%)	15.6
ICE MILK (VANILLA, 4% FAT)	26.4
IMITATION CREAMER (POWDERED)	2000.0
IMITATION SOUR DRESSING	37.1
IMITATION WHIPPED TOPING	2000.0
ITALIAN BREAD	12.8
ITALIAN SALAD DRESSING (LOW CAL)	400.0
ITALIAN SALAD DRESSING (REGULAR)	200.0
JAMS AND FRUIT PRESERVES	20000.0
JELLY BEANS	52000.0
JERUSALEM-ARTICHOKE	13.0
KIWIFRUIT	22.0
LEMON JUICE	32.0
LEMON MERINGUE PIE	24.6
LEMONADE	42000.0
LEMON-LIME SODA	78000.0
LEMONS (RAW)	10.0
LUCKY CHARMS CEREAL	15.3
MACARONI	11.1
MACARONI AND CHEESE	11.4
MALTED MILK (CHOCOLATE)	16.4
MALTED MILK (REGULAR)	14.9

MALT-O-MEAL	13.0
MANGO (RAW)	70.0
MARSHMALLOWS	46.0
MAYONNAISE (IMITATION)	4000.0
MAYONNAISE SALAD DRESSING	8000.0
MILK (WHOLE)	13.3
MOLASSES	44000.0
NATURE VALLEY GRANOLA CEREAL	21.2
NECTARINES	32.0
OATMEAL & RAISIN COOKIES	24.2
OATMEAL (FLAVORED)	12.4
OATMEAL BREAD	11.3
ONION RINGS	16.2
ONIONS (RAW)	12.0
ORANGE & GRAPEFRUIT JUICE	50.0
ORANGE (RAW)	30.0
ORANGE JUICE (CANNED)	50.0
ORANGE JUICE (FRESH)	26.0
ORANGE SODA	92000.0
PANCAKES (BUCKWHEAT)	12.0
PANCAKES (PLAIN)	16.0
PAPAYA	34.0
PARMESAN CHEESE	15.4
PARSNIPS	22.5
PEACH PIE	33.1
PEACHES (CANNED, HEAVY SYRUP)	102.0
PEACHES (CANNED, JUICE)	29.0
PEACHES (DRIED)	32.7
PEACHES (FRESH)	20.0
PEANUT BUTTER COOKIE	16.7
PEAR (CANNED, HEAVY SYRUP)	98.0

PEAR (CANNED, JUICE)	64.0
PEAR (FRESH)	37.5
PECAN PIE	38.3
PICKLES (CUCUMBER)	600.0
PICKLES (CUCUMBER, DILL)	200.0
PICKLES (CUCUMBER, SWEET)	1000.0
PIE CRUST	17.1
PINEAPPLE (CANNED, HEAVY SYRUP)	104.0
PINEAPPLE (CANNED, JUICE)	78.0
PINEAPPLE (FRESH)	38.0
PINEAPPLE JUICE (UNSWEETENED)	68.0
PINEAPPLE-GRAPEFRUIT JUICE DRINK	46000.0
PITA BREAD	11.0
PIZZA (CHEESE)	10.9
PLANTAINS	42.8
PLUMS (CANNED, HEAVY SYRUP)	120.0
PLUMS (CANNED, JUICE)	76.0
PLUMS (FRESH)	18.0
POPCORN (SYRUP)	22.5
POPSICLE	36000.0
POTATO CHIPS	20.1
POTATOES (AU GRATIN)	23.7
POTATOES (BAKED, NO SKIN)	22.7
POTATOES (BAKED, WITH SKIN)	20.4
POTATOES (BOILED)	18.0
POTATOES (FRENCH FRIES, BAKED)	20.8
POTATOES (FRENCH FRIES, FRIED)	20.2
POTATOES (HASHED BROWN)	22.6
POTATOES (MASHED)	26.7
POTATOES (SCALLOPED)	22.4
POUND CAKE	31.7

PRETZELS	13.0
PRODUCT 19 CEREAL	16.0
PRUNE JUICE	22.5
PRUNES (DRIED)	31.0
PUMPERNICKEL BREAD	10.7
PUMPKIN (CANNED)	13.3
PUMPKIN (FRESH)	12.0
PUMPKIN PIE	18.4
QUICHE LORRAINE	13.1
RADISHES	200.0
RAISIN BRAN CEREAL	10.5
RAISIN BREAD	13.0
RAISINS	34.5
RASPBERRIES (SWEETENED)	55.5
RELISH (SWEET)	100.0
RHUBARB (SWEETENED)	150.0
RICE (BROWN)	20.0
RICE (WHITE)	25.0
RICE KRISPIES CEREAL	25.0
RICE PUDDING	18.3
RICOTTA CHEESE (SKIM MILK)	15.0
RICOTTA CHEESE (WHOLE MILK)	15.9
ROLLS (DINNER)	28.0
ROLLS (FRANKFURTER & HAMBURGER)	13.3
ROLLS (HARD)	12.0
ROLLS (HOAGIE OR SUBMARINE)	13.2
ROOT BEER	84000.0
RYE WAFERS (WHOLE-GRAIN)	15.0
SALTINES	18.0
SEAWEED (KELP)	60.0
SELF-RISING FLOUR (UNSIFTED)	15.5

SEMI SWEET CHOCOLATE	41.3
SHEETCAKE (NO FROSTING)	29.9
SHEETCAKE (WHITE FROSTING)	54.8
SHERBET	69.0
SHORTBREAD COOKIE	210.0
SHREDDED WHEAT CEREAL	11.5
SNACK CAKES (DEVIL'S FOOD & CRÈME)	36.1
SNACK CAKES (SPONGE & CRÈME)	57.5
SOUR CREAM	18.2
SPAGHETTI (SOFT)	12.8
SPAGHETTI (TOMATO SAUCE, CHEESE)	13.0
SQUASH (WINTER)	18.0
STRAWBERRIES (FRESH)	15.0
STRAWBERRIES (FROZEN, SWEETENED)	55.5
SUGAR (BROWN)	424000.0
SUGAR (WHITE)	398000.0
SUGAR COOKIE	31.1
SUGAR SMACKS CEREAL	25.0
SUPER SUGAR CRISP CEREAL	26.0
SWEET POTATOE PIE	58000.2
SWEET POTATOES (BAKED)	21.0
SWEETPOTATOES (CANNED)	12.0
SWEETPOTATOES (CANNED, MASHED)	23.6
SWISS CHEESE	10.3
SWISS CHEESE	10.3
SYRUP (LIGHT, CHOCOLATE FLAVORED)	44.0
SYRUP (CORN, MAPLE)	64000.0
SYRUP (THICK, CHOCOLATE FLAVORED)	28.2
TANGERINE JUICE	60.0
TANGERINES (CANNED, LIGHT SYRUP)	82.0
TANGERINES (FRESH)	18.0

TAPIOCA PUDDING	50.4
TARTAR SAUCE	200.0
THOUSAND ISLAND DRESSING	400.0
TOASTER PASTRIES	38.1
TOMATO & VEGETABLE SOUP	12.0
TOMATO JUICE	10.0
TOMATO PASTE	10.9
TOMATO PUREE	12.5
TOMATO SOUP (MILK)	11.9
TOMATO SOUP (WATER)	17.0
TOMATOES (CANNED)	10.0
TOTAL CEREAL	14.7
TRIX CEREAL	25.0
TURNIPS	16.0
VANILLA PUDDING	89.7
VANILLA SHAKE	18.2
VANILLA WAFERS	29.1
VIENNA BREAD	13.0
WAFFLES	10.4
WATER CHESTNUTS	34.0
WATERMELON	23.3
WHEAT BREAD	10.3
WHEAT CRACKERS	10.0
WHEAT FLOUR (ALL-PURPOSE, SIFTED	14.7
WHEAT FLOUR (ALL-PURPOSE, UNSIFTED)	14.6
WHEATIES CEREAL	15.3
WHIPPED TOPPING	19.8
WHIPPING CREAM (HEAVY)	18.5
WHIPPING CREAM (LIGHT)	18.5
WHITE BREAD	15.4
WHITE BREAD CRUMBS	11.0

WHITE BREAD CUBES	15.0
WHITE CAKE (WHITE FROSTING)	34.0
WHITE SAUCE (MILK)	11.3
WHOLE-WHEAT BREAD	10.4
YELLOW CAKE (CHOCOLATE FROSTING)	35.0
YOGURT (FRUIT, LOW FAT MILK)	12.9
YOGURT (WHOLE MILK)	14.7

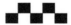

FP 'GREEN' TABLE

Eat foods from this table for 2 weeks along with foods from the FP 'Yellow' table.

Name of food	FP value
BRAN FLAKES (40%)	0.0
ALFALFA SEEDS (SPROUTED, RAW)	0.0
ALL-BRAN CEREAL	1.1
ANGELFOOD CAKE	0.2
APPLES (DRIED, SULFURED)	0.0
APRICOT (CANNED, HEAVY SYRUP)	0.0
APRICOT NECTAR	0.0
APRICOTS (CANNED, IN JUICE)	0.0
APRICOTS (DRIED)	0.0
APRICOTS (RAW)	0.0
ARTICHOKES (GLOBE, COOKED)	0.0
ASPARAGUS (CANNED)	0.0
ASPARAGUS (FROZEN)	0.0
BAGELS (EGG)	1.3
BAGELS (PLAIN)	1.3
BARLEY (PEARLED, LIGHT)	0.6
BEAN SPROUTS	0.0
BEEF HEART (BRAISED)	1.0
BEEF ROAST (LEAN, EYE O RND)	1.2
BEER (LIGHT)	0.0
BEER (REGULAR)	0.0
BEET GREENS	0.0
BEETS (CANNED)	0.0
BEETS (COOKED, DRAINED)	0.0
BLACK BEANS (COOKED, DRAINED)	0.3

BLACK-EYED PEAS, DRY, COOKED	0.4
BLUEBERRIES (FROZEN, SWEETENED)	0.0
BROCCOLI (FROZEN, COOKED, DRAINED)	0.0
BROCCOLI (RAW, COOKED, DRAINED)	0.0
BRUSSELS SPROUTS	0.8
BUCKWHEAT FLOUR (LIGHT, SIFTED)	0.8
BULGUR	0.8
CABBAGE (CHINESE)	0.0
CABBAGE (COMMON)	0.0
CABBAGE (RED)	0.0
CABBAGE (SAVOY)	0.0
CAKE & PASTRY FLOUR	0.6
CAROB FLOUR	0.0
CARROTS (FROZEN, COOKED)	0.0
CARROTS (RAW)	0.0
CATSUP	0.9
CAULIFLOWER	0.0
CELERY (PASCAL, RAW)	0.0
CHERRIES (SOUR, CANNED, WATER)	0.0
CHICKEN (LIGHT & DARK, STEWED)	1.3
CHICKEN BREAST (ROASTED)	0.5
CHICKEN CHOW MEIN	0.0
CHICKEN DRUMSTICK (ROASTED)	0.8
CHICKEN LIVER	0.9
CHICKPEAS	1.3
CLAMS	0.4
COLLARDS	0.0
CORN (CREAM, CANNED)	1.1
CORN FLAKES	1.0
CORN GRITS (WHITE)	0.0
CORN GRITS (YELLOW)	0.0

COTTAGE CHEESE (UNCREAMED)	0.2
CRABMEAT	0.6
CRANBERRY SAUCE (SWEATENED, CANNED)	0.0
CREAM OF WHEAT	1.0
DATES	1.1
EGG NOODLES	1.3
EGGPLANT	0.0
EGGS (WHITE, RAW)	0.0
ENGLISH MUFFINS (PLAIN)	0.9
EVAPORATED MILK (NONFAT)	0.2
FLOUNDER (BAKED, NO FAT)	0.3
FROSTED FLAKES CEREAL	1.0
FRUIT COCKTAIL (CANNED, HEAVY SYRUP)	0.0
FRUIT COCKTAIL (CANNED, JUICE)	0.0
GELATIN DESSERT	1.0
GRAPE JUICE (CANNED)	1.0
GRAPEFRUIT (CANNED, SYRUP)	0.0
GRAPEFRUIT (RAW)	0.0
GRAPEFRUIT JUICE (SWEETENED)	1.0
GRAPEFRUIT JUICE (UNSWEETENED)	0.0
GRAPE-NUTS CEREAL	0.5
GREAT NORTHERN BEANS (DRY, DRAINED)	0.3
HONEY	1.0
HONEYDEW MELON	0.0
ITALIAN BREAD	0.5
JERUSALEM-ARTICHOKE	0.0
KALE	1.1
KIWIFRUIT	0.0

KOHLRABI	0.0
LEMONS (RAW)	0.0
LENTILS	0.3
LETTUCE (BUTTER-HEAD)	0.0
LETTUCE (CRISP-HEAD)	0.9
LETTUCE (LOOSE LEAF)	0.0
LIMA BEANS	0.3
MACARONI	0.6
MALT-O-MEAL	0.0
MARSHMALLOWS	0.0
MELBA TOAST	0.0
MILK (SKIM)	0.5
MUSHROOMS (CANNED)	0.0
MUSHROOMS (RAW)	0.0
MUSTARD GREENS	0.0
NONFAT DRY MILK	0.1
OKRA	0.0
ONION SOUP	0.0
ONIONS (RAW)	0.0
ONIONS (RAW, SPRING)	0.0
ORANGE & GRAPEFRUIT JUICE	0.5
ORANGE (RAW)	0.0
ORANGE JUICE (CANNED)	0.5
ORANGE JUICE (FRESH)	0.5
OYSTERS (RAW)	1.0
PAPAYA	0.0
PARSNIPS	0.0
PEA BEANS (DRY)	0.3
PEACHES (CANNED, HEAVY SYRUP)	0.0
PEACHES (CANNED, JUICE)	0.0
PEACHES (DRIED)	0.8

PEACHES (FRESH)	0.0
PEAR (CANNED, HEAVY SYRUP)	0.0
PEAR (CANNED, JUICE)	0.0
PEAS (CANNED, GREEN)	0.6
PEAS (FRESH, GREEN)	0.1
PEAS (POD)	0.0
PEPPERS (HOT GREEN CHILI)	0.0
PEPPERS (HOT RED CHILI)	0.0
PEPPERS (SWEET GREEN)	0.0
PEPPERS (SWEET RED)	0.0
PINEAPPLE (CANNED, HEAVY SYRUP)	0.0
PINEAPPLE (CANNED, JUICE)	0.0
PINEAPPLE JUICE (UNSWEETENED)	0.0
PINTO BEANS	0.3
PITA BREAD	0.8
PLANTAINS	0.0
PLUMS (CANNED, HEAVY SYRUP)	0.0
PLUMS (CANNED, JUICE)	0.0
PLUMS (FRESH)	0.0
POPCORN (AIR-POPPED)	0.0
PORK (CURED, HAM, LEAN)	1.1
PORK (LUNCHEON MEAT, HAM, LEAN)	1.2
POTATOES (BAKED, NO SKIN)	0.0
POTATOES (BAKED, WITH SKIN)	0.0
POTATOES (BOILED)	0.0
PRODUCT 19 CEREAL	1.0
PRUNE JUICE	0.0
PRUNES (DRIED)	0.0
PUMPKIN (FRESH)	0.0
RAISINS	0.9
RASPBERRIES (SWEETENED)	0.5

RED KIDNEY BEANS	0.3
REFRIED BEANS	0.8
RHUBARB (SWEETENED)	0.0
RICE (BROWN)	0.9
RICE (WHITE)	0.0
RICE KRISPIES CEREAL	0.0
SALMON (CANNED)	1.3
SALMON (RED, BAKED)	1.1
SAUERKRAUT	0.0
SEAWEED (SPIRULINA)	0.6
SELF-RISING FLOUR (UNSIFTED)	0.4
SHRIMP	0.2
SNAP BEAN (GREEN)	0.0
SNAP BEAN (YELLOW)	0.0
SOLE (BAKED, NO FAT)	0.3
SOY SAUCE	0.0
SPAGHETTI (FIRM)	0.6
SPAGHETTI (SOFT)	0.9
SPECIAL K CEREAL	0.0
SPINACH (CANNED)	0.8
SPINACH (FRESH)	0.0
SPINACH (FROZEN)	0.0
SUPER SUGAR CRISP CEREAL	0.0
SWEET POTATOES (BAKED)	0.0
SWEETPOTATOES (CANNED)	0.0
SWEETPOTATOES (CANNED, MASHED)	0.9
SYRUP (LIGHT, CHOCOLATE FLAVORED)	0.0
TANGERINE JUICE	1.0
TANGERINES (CANNED, LIGHT SYRUP)	0.0
TANGERINES (FRESH)	0.0
TOMATO JUICE	0.0

TOMATO PASTE	1.0
TOMATO PUREE	0.0
TOMATOES (FRESH)	0.0
TRIX CEREAL	1.0
TUNA (CANNED, LIGHT, OIL, DRAINNED)	1.4
TUNA (CANNED, LIGHT, WATER)	0.2
TURKEY (LIGHT & DARK, ROASTED)	1.0
TURKEY (ROASTED)	0.5
TURKEY HAM (CURED)	1.2
TURKEY LOAF	0.5
TURNIP GREENS (FRESH)	0.0
TURNIP GREENS (FROZEN)	0.9
TURNIPS	0.0
VEGETABLE JUICE	0.0
VEGETABLES (MIXED)	0.0
WATER CHESTNUTS	0.0
WHEAT FLOUR (ALL-PURPOSE, SIFTED	0.4
WHEAT FLOUR (ALL-PURPOSE, UNSIFTED)	0.3
WHEATIES CEREAL	1.0
WHOLE-WHEAT FLOUR	0.6
YOGURT (NONFAT MILK)	0.0

FP 'YELLOW' TABLE

Eat foods from this table for 2 weeks along with foods from the FP 'Green' table.

Name of food	FP value
BAMBOO SHOOTS (CANNED)	2.3
BEEF BROTH (BOULLION)	1.5
BEEF NOODLE SOUP	2.7
BOSTON BROWN BREAD	2.3
BREADCRUMBS	1.8
BROWN GRAVY (DRY MIX)	3.0
CANTALOUP	2.3
CHEERIOS CEREAL	2.3
CHESTNUTS (ROASTED)	2.7
CHICKEN (CANNED)	1.8
CHICKEN BREAST (FRIED VEG OIL, FLOUR)	1.5
CHICKEN DRUMSTICK, (FRD VEG OIL, FLOUR)	2.6
CHICKEN GRAVY (DRY MIX)	3.0
CHICKEN NOODLE SOUP	2.3
CHICKEN RICE SOUP	2.3
CHICKEN ROLL	1.8
CHOCOLATE MILK (LOWFAT 1%)	1.9
CLAM CHOWDER (MANHATTAN)	2.3
COCOA POWDER (NONFAT DRY MILK)	1.5
CORN (RAW, WHITE)	1.5
CORN (RAW, YELLOW)	2.3
CORNMEAL	2.0
CRACKED-WHEAT BREAD	2.3

CRACKED-WHEAT BREAD	1.9
DANDELION GREENS	2.3
FIGS (DRIED)	1.5
FISH STICKS	2.3
FLOUNDER (BAKED IN VEG OIL)	1.7
FRENCH BREAD	2.1
FROOT LOOPS CEREAL	2.3
GOLDEN GRAHAMS CEREAL	2.3
GREEN PEAS (SOUP)	1.7
HADDOCK (BREADED, FRIED VEG OIL)	2.6
HONEY NUT CHEERIOS CEREAL	1.5
LUCKY CHARMS CEREAL	1.5
MISO	2.2
MIXED GRAIN BREAD	1.8
OATMEAL (FLAVORED)	1.8
OATMEAL (PLAIN)	2.3
OATMEAL BREAD	2.5
POPCORN (SYRUP)	2.3
PRETZELS	2.3
PUMPERNICKEL BREAD	1.9
PUMPKIN (CANNED)	1.5
RAISIN BRAN CEREAL	1.5
RAISIN BREAD	2.3
ROLLS (FRANKFURTER & HAMBURGER)	3.0
ROLLS (HARD)	1.8
RYE BREAD (LIGHT)	2.2
SARDINES (CANNED, OIL, ATLANTIC)	2.2
SHREDDED WHEAT CEREAL	1.5
SHRIMP (FRIED, NOT BREADED, NOT BATTERED)	3.0
SOLE (BAKED IN VEG OIL)	1.7

SOYBEANS	2.4
SPAGHETTI (TOMATO SAUCE)	1.5
SQUASH (SUMMER)	2.3
SQUASH (WINTER)	2.3
SUGAR SMACKS CEREAL	2.3
TOFU	2.5
TOMATOES (CANNED)	2.3
TORTILLAS (CORN)	2.3
TOTAL CEREAL	1.5
TUNA SALAD	2.7
TURKEY AND GRAVY	2.6
VEGETABLE & BEEF SOUP	1.5
VIENNA BREAD	2.3
WATERMELON	3.0
WHEAT BREAD	2.2
WHITE BREAD CRUMBS	2.3
WHITE BREAD CUBES	2.3

FP 'RED' TABLE

Avoid the foods in this table during this 2 week rotation

Name of food	FP value
ALMONDS (SLIVERED)	11.8
AMERICAN CHEESE	18.6
AMERICAN CHEESE SPREAD	14.2
APPLE JUICE (CANNED)	4.5
APPLE PIE	25.9
APPLE PIE (FRIED)	36.7
APPLES (RAW, UNPEELED)	4.5
APPLESAUCE (CANNED, SWEETENED)	4.5
APPLESAUCE (CANNED,UNSWEETENED)	4.5
AVOCADOS (CALIFORNIA)	33.9
AVOCADOS (FLORIDA)	24.5
BANANAS	4.5
BARBECUE SAUCE	4.5
BEAN WITH BACON SOUP	3.5
BEANS (CANNED, FRANKFURTER)	9.8
BEANS (PORK, SWEET SAUCE)	7.2
BEANS (PORK, TOMATO SAUCE)	4.5
BEEF (DRIED)	3.3
BEEF (LEAN & FAT CHUCK BLADE)	11.3
BEEF (LEAN & FAT, BOTTOM ROUND)	6.5
BEEF (LEAN, BOTTOM ROUND)	4.1
BEEF (LEAN, CHUCK BLADE)	6.9
BEEF AND VEGETABLE STEW	7.6
BEEF GRAVY	7.7
BEEF LIVER (FRIED)	4.1
BEEF POTPIE	9.4
BEEF ROAST (LEAN & FAT, EYE O RND)	7.1

BEEF ROAST (LEAN & FAT, RIBS)	12.2
BEEF ROAST (LEAN, RIBS)	6.5
BEEF STEAK (LEAN, SIRLOIN, BROIL)	4.8
BISCUIT BAKING MIX	6.8
BLACKBERRIES (RAW)	4.5
BLUE CHEESE	17.6
BLUE CHEESE SALAD DRESSING	36.1
BLUEBERRIES (RAW)	4.5
BLUEBERRY MUFFINS	7.6
BLUEBERRY PIE	23.2
BOLOGNA	15.0
BOUILLON (DEHYDRATED)	4.5
BRAN MUFFINS	6.1
BRAUNSCHWEIGER	14.2
BRAZIL NUTS	21.6
BREAD STUFFING (DRY MIX)	15.7
BROWNIES WITH NUTS	27.1
BUTTER	429.6
BUTTERMILK (DRIED)	9.7
CAMEMBERT CHEESE	16.5
CANDY (MILK CHOCOLATE, ALMONDS)	21.1
CANDY (MILK CHOCOLATE, PEANUTS)	16.5
CANDY (MILK CHOCOLATE, PLAIN)	29.9
CANDY (MILK CHOCOLATE, RICE CRISPIES)	25.2
CAP'N CRUNCH CEREAL	16.5
CARAMEL	20.2
CARROT CAKE (CREME CHESE FROSTING)	25.9
CASHEW NUTS (DRY ROASTD)	14.8
CASHEW NUTS (ROASTED, OIL)	13.7
CELERY SEED	4.5
CEREAL (100% NATURAL)	19.7

CHEDDAR CHEESE	18.3
CHEESE CRACKERS (PEANUT SANDWICH)	9.0
CHEESE CRACKERS (PLAIN)	4.5
CHEESE SAUCE WITH MILK	14.3
CHEESEBURGER	11.7
CHEESECAKE	29.7
CHERRIES (RAW, SWEET)	4.5
CHERRY PIE	22.7
CHERRY PIE (FRIED)	36.7
CHICKEN A LA KING	11.3
CHICKEN AND NOODLES	6.6
CHICKEN BREAST (FRIED, BATTERED)	5.1
CHICKEN DRUMSTICK (FRIED, BATTERED)	5.5
CHICKEN FRANKFURTER	7.0
CHICKEN GRAVY (CANNED)	12.8
CHICKEN POTPIE	10.6
CHILI	8.1
CHOCOLATE (SWEET, DARK)	54.6
CHOCOLATE (FOR BAKING, BITTER)	33.9
CHOCOLATE CHIP COOKIES	23.0
CHOCOLATE MILK (LOWFAT 2%)	10.0
CHOCOLATE MILK (REGULAR)	15.7
CHOCOLATE PUDDING	9.3
CHOCOLATE SHAKE	13.5
CHOP SUEY (BEEF & PORK)	5.5
CHOW MEIN NOODLES	8.4
CLAM CHOWDER (NEW ENGLAND, MILK)	7.5
CLUB SODA	4.5
COCOA POWDER (REGULAR)	14.1
COCONUT (RAW)	115.2
COCONUT (SHREDDED, DRIED,	109.7

SWEETENED)	
COFFEE	4.5
COFFEE CREAM (LIGHT)	49.8
COFFEECAKE (CRUMB)	10.4
COLA (DIET)	4.5
COLA (REGULAR)	4.5
CONDENSED MILK (SWEETENED)	19.2
CORN CHIPS	20.3
CORN MUFFINS	7.6
CORN OIL	981000.1
CORNED BEEF (CANNED)	6.7
COTTAGE CHEESE (FRUIT)	11.2
COTTAGE CHEESE (LARGE CURDS, CREAMED)	13.3
COTTAGE CHEESE (LOWFAT 2%)	8.8
CRACKERS (SNACK)	4500.0
CRANBERRY JUICE COCKTAL	4.5
CREAM CHEESE	33.3
CREAM OF CHICKEN SOUP (MILK)	12.0
CREAM OF CHICKEN SOUP (WATER)	10.7
CREAM OF MUSHROM SOUP (MILK)	14.6
CREAM OF MUSHROOM SOUP (WATER)	20.4
CREME PIE	49.2
CROISSANTS	13.4
CUCUMBER (WITH PEEL)	4.5
CUSTARD (BAKED)	11.5
CUSTARD PIE	13.5
DANISH PASTRY (FRUIT)	17.5
DANISH PASTRY (PLAIN)	19.3
DEVIL'S FOOD CAKE (CHOCOLATE FROSTING)	20.3

DOUGHNUTS (CAKE TYPE, PLAIN)	18.2
DOUGHNUTS (YEAST-LEAVENED, GLAZED)	24.3
DUCK (ROASTED)	7.2
EGG NOG	21.3
EGGS (FRIED)	5.4
EGGS (HARD-BOILED)	3.9
EGGS (POACHED)	3.9
EGGS (SCRAMBLED)	4.7
EGGS (WHOLE, RAW)	3.9
EGGS (YOLK, RAW)	7.6
ENCHILADA	10.8
ENG MUFFIN (BACON, EGG, CHEESE)	10.9
EVAPORATED MILK (WHOLE)	17.6
FETA CHEESE	18.2
FIG BARS	9.0
FILBERTS (HAZELNUTS)	21.7
FISH SANDWICH (CHEESE)	9.5
FISH SANDWICH (NO CHEESE)	9.2
FLOUNDER (BAKED IN BUTTER)	7.5
FRANKFURTER	15.8
FRENCH SALAD DRESSING (LOW CAL)	9000.0
FRENCH SALAD DRESSING (REGULAR)	40500.0
FRENCH TOAST	5.3
FRUIT JELLIES	4.5
FRUIT PUNCH DRINK (CANNED)	4.5
FRUITCAKE	16.5
FUDGE, CHOCOLATE, PLAIN	20.5
GINGER ALE	4.5
GINGERBREAD CAKE	12.6
GRAHAM CRACKER (PLAIN)	4.5
GRAPE DRINK (CANNED)	4.5

GRAPE SODA	4.5
GRAPES (RAW)	4.5
GROUND BEEF (BROILED, LEAN & FAT)	9.0
GROUND BEEF (BROILED, LEAN)	8.2
GUM DROPS	4.5
HALF AND HALF (CREAM)	31.9
HALIBUT (BROILED, BUTTER & LEMON JUICE)	7.6
HAMBURGER	8.6
HARD CANDY	4.5
HERRING (PICKLED)	6.8
HOLLANDAISE (WATER)	29.3
ICE CREAM (VANLLA,11% FAT)	29.3
ICE CREAM (VANLLA,16% FAT)	42.0
ICE MILK (VANILLA, 3%)	8.9
ICE MILK (VANILLA, 4% FAT)	20.0
IMITATION CREAMER (POWDERED)	4500.0
IMITATION SOUR DRESSING	56.2
IMITATION WHIPPED TOPING	3600.0
ITALIAN SALAD DRESSING (LOW CAL)	4.5
ITALIAN SALAD DRESSING (REGULAR)	40500.0
JAMS AND FRUIT PRESERVES	4.5
JELLY BEANS	4.5
LAMB (LEG, LEAN & FAT, ROASTED)	8.2
LAMB (LEG, LEAN, ROASTED)	4.4
LAMB CHOPS (ARM, LEAN & FAT, BRAISED)	9.9
LAMB CHOPS (ARM, LEAN, BRAISED)	5.7
LAMB CHOPS (LOIN, LEAN & FAT, BROIL)	9.8
LAMB CHOPS (LOIN, LEAN, BROIL)	5.0
LAMB RIB (LEAN & FAT, ROASTED)	13.9
LAMB RIB (LEAN, ROASTED)	6.7

LARD	922506.3
LEMON JUICE	4.5
LEMON MERINGUE PIE	16.6
LEMONADE	4.5
LEMON-LIME SODA	4.5
LIQUOR (GIN, RUM, VODKA, WHISKY, COGNAC...)	4.5
MACADAMIA NUTS (OIL ROASTED)	46.5
MACARONI AND CHEESE	12.5
MALTED MILK (CHOCOLATE)	14.5
MALTED MILK (REGULAR)	14.1
MANGO (RAW)	4.5
MARGARINE (REGULAR, HARD)	49500.1
MARGARINE (IMITATION 40% FAT)	396.2
MARGARINE (REGULAR, HARD, 80% FAT)	409.7
MARGARINE (REGULR, SOFT)	49500.1
MARGARINE (REGULR, SOFT, 80% FAT)	823.7
MARGARINE (SPREAD, HARD, 60% FAT)	313.3
MARGARINE (SPREAD, SOFT, 60% FAT)	623.6
MAYONNAISE (IMITATION)	13500.0
MAYONNAISE (REGULAR)	49500.1
MAYONNAISE SALAD DRESSING	22500.0
MILK (1% LOW FAT)	4.4
MILK (2% LOW FAT)	8.6
MILK (WHOLE)	15.0
MINESTRONE SOUP	3.4
MIXED NUTS (DRY ROASTED, NO HONEY)	16.9
MIXED NUTS (OIL ROASTED, NO HONEY)	14.5
MOLASSES	4.5
MOZZARELLA CHEESE (WHOLE MILK)	12.7
MOZZARELLA CHESE (SKIM MILK)	10.0

MUENSTER CHEESE	15.4
MUSHROOM GRAVY	9.0
MUSTARD (YELLOW)	4.5
NATURE VALLEY GRANOLA CEREAL	16.0
NECTARINES	4.5
OATMEAL & RAISIN COOKIES	15.2
OCEAN PERCH (FRIED, BREADED)	3.3
OLIVE OIL	972000.2
OLIVES (BLACK)	9000.0
OLIVES (GREEN)	9000.0
ONION RINGS	22.7
ORANGE SODA	4.5
OYSTERS (FRIED, BREADED)	4.6
PANCAKES (BUCKWHEAT)	4.5
PANCAKES (PLAIN)	4.5
PARMESAN CHEESE	18.4
PARMESAN CHEESE	13.3
PEACH PIE	21.9
PEANUT BUTTER	7.3
PEANUT BUTTER COOKIE	18.5
PEANUT OIL	972000.2
PEANUTS (OIL-ROASTED)	7.9
PEAR (FRESH)	4.5
PECAN PIE	22.7
PECANS (HALVES)	41.1
PICKLES (CUCUMBER)	4.5
PICKLES (CUCUMBER, DILL)	4.5
PICKLES (CUCUMBER, SWEET)	4.5
PIE CRUST	23.9
PINE NUTS	38.4
PINEAPPLE (FRESH)	4.5

PINEAPPLE-GRAPEFRUIT JUICE DRINK	4.5
PISTACHIO NUTS	10.6
PIZZA (CHEESE)	8.2
POPCORN (VEGETABLE OIL)	13.5
POPSICLE	4.5
PORK (CURED, BACON)	10.2
PORK (CURED, HAM, LEAN & FAT)	7.8
PORK (LINK)	6.1
PORK (LUNCHEON MEAT, CANNED)	15.4
PORK (ROASTED HAM, LEAN)	4.5
PORK CHOP LOIN (BROILED, LEAN & FAT)	8.3
PORK CHOP LOIN (BROILED, LEAN)	4.1
PORK CHOP LOIN (FRIED, LEAN & FAT)	10.6
PORK CHOP LOIN (FRIED, LEAN)	6.1
PORK FRESH (ROASTED HAM, LEAN & FAT)	8.4
PORK RIBS (ROASTED, LEAN & FAT)	8.8
PORK RIBS (ROASTED, LEAN)	5.5
PORK SHOULDER (BRAISED, LEAN & FAT)	8.9
PORK SHOULDER (BRAISED, LEAN)	4.5
POTATO CHIPS	31.6
POTATO SALAD (MAYONNAISE)	13.6
POTATOES (AU GRATIN)	20.3
POTATOES (FRENCH FRIES, BAKED)	12.8
POTATOES (FRENCH FRIES, FRIED)	18.2
POTATOES (HASHED BROWN)	21.2
POTATOES (MASHED)	24.2
POTATOES (SCALLOPED)	19.9
POUND CAKE	28.2
PROVOLONE CHEESE	14.1
PUMPKIN AND SQUASH KERNELS	8.5
PUMPKIN PIE	18.8

QUICHE LORRAINE	25.2
RADISHES	4.5
RELISH (SWEET)	4.5
RICE PUDDING	9.3
RICOTTA CHEESE (SKIM MILK)	17.2
RICOTTA CHEESE (WHOLE MILK)	20.5
ROAST BEEF SANDWICH	5.1
ROLLS (DINNER)	9.0
ROLLS (HOAGIE OR SUBMARINE)	3.4
ROOT BEER	4.5
RYE WAFERS (WHOLE-GRAIN)	4.5
SAFFLOWER OIL	981000.1
SALAMI (DRY)	8.8
SALAMI (NOT DRY)	11.1
SALMON (SMOKED)	4.5
SALTINES	4.5
SANDWICH SPREAD (BEEF & PORK)	13.5
SAUSAGE (BROWN AND SERVE)	11.4
SCALLOPS (BREADED)	3.2
SEAWEED (KELP)	4.5
SEMI SWEET CHOCOLATE	52.8
SESAME SEEDS	9.0
SHEETCAKE (NO FROSTING)	18.3
SHEETCAKE (WHITE FROSTING)	24.5
SHERBET	22.0
SHORTBREAD COOKIE	194.5
SNACK CAKES (DEVIL'S FOOD & CRÈME)	20.1
SNACK CAKES (SPONGE & CRÈME)	26.0
SOLE (BAKED IN BUTTER)	7.5
SOUR CREAM	46.2
SOYBEAN OIL (HYDROGENATED)	981000.2

SOYBEAN-COTTONSEED OIL (HYDROGENATED)	981000.2
SPAGHETTI (MEATBALLS, TOMATO SAUCE)	3.9
SPINACH SOUFFLE	12.5
STEAK (BROILED, SIRLOIN)	8.5
STRAWBERRIES (FRESH)	4.5
STRAWBERRIES (FROZEN, SWEETENED)	4.5
SUGAR (BROWN)	4.5
SUGAR (WHITE)	4.5
SUGAR COOKIE	27.1
SUNFLOWER OIL	981000.1
SUNFLOWER SEEDS	10.5
SWEET POTATOE PIE	13500.2
SWISS CHEESE	14.5
SWISS CHEESE	14.5
SYRUP (CORN, MAPLE)	4.5
SYRUP (THICK, CHOCOLATE FLAVORED)	18.5
TACO	9.4
TAHINI	12.0
TAPIOCA PUDDING	39.2
TARTAR SAUCE	36000.0
TEA (BREWED, UNSWEETENED)	4.5
THOUSAND ISLAND DRESSING	27000.0
TOASTER PASTRIES	13.6
TOMATO & VEGETABLE SOUP	4.5
TOMATO SOUP (MILK)	9.1
TOMATO SOUP (WATER)	4.5
TROUT (BROILED, BUTTER)	7.2
TURKEY PATTIES (BATTERED, FRIED)	8.0
VANILLA PUDDING	79.2
VANILLA SHAKE	12.8

VANILLA WAFERS	15.9
VEAL CUTLET (BROILED, ROASTED, BRAISED)	7.1
VEAL RIB (BROILED, ROASTED, BRAISED)	8.3
VEGETARIAN SOUP	4.5
VIENNA SAUSAGE	9.1
VINEGAR AND OIL SALAD DRESSING	36000.1
WAFFLES	7.8
WALNUTS (BLACK)	10.3
WALNUTS (ENGLISH)	19.7
WHEAT CRACKERS	4.5
WHIPPED TOPPING	42.1
WHIPPING CREAM (HEAVY)	94.9
WHIPPING CREAM (LIGHT)	82.3
WHITE BREAD	5.6
WHITE CAKE (WHITE FROSTING)	18.3
WHITE SAUCE (MILK)	13.0
WHOLE-WHEAT BREAD	5.3
WHOLE-WHEAT WAFERS	9.0
YELLOW CAKE (CHOCOLATE FROSTING)	18.8
YOGURT (FRUIT, LOW FAT MILK)	5.2
YOGURT (PLAIN, LOW FAT MILK)	6.3
YOGURT (WHOLE MILK)	15.8

--------------- *Chapter Six* ---------------

Ready, Set, Go!!!

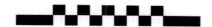

Now, you have good knowledge of what you need to do to enjoy a rapid and complete weight loss with the clinique science weight loss system. I would like however, to use the next few pages to summarize the system, so that it is easier for you to apply this knowledge. As you read this chapter, I would like you to take notes on everything that concerns your weight and your health – e.g. your BMI, the food content in your kitchen, your eating habits, your level of activity, your level of commitment to the clinique science weight loss system, your weight loss goal(s), your level of belief in yourself, etc.

About food – what, when, and how?

<u>The facts</u>
- Eating medicinal foods everyday will greatly improve your health and facilitate your weight loss.
- Some foods such as nuts (almonds, peanuts, pecans, and walnuts) and dark cocoa may contribute directly to your weight loss through a series of therapeutic mechanisms.
- It doesn't matter when you eat. It is however beneficial to eat breakfast followed by several small meals throughout the day.
- When you become overweight or obese, your body does not process carbohydrates and fats efficiently. It has a tendency to store both the carbohydrates and fats that you eat as fat in the fat cells of your body – making you even fatter. The body however continues to process proteins efficiently. As a matter of fact, if you eat the right kind of proteins while eliminating certain carbohydrates and fats from your diet, you will lose weight.
- You lose weight faster, and lose more weight, when you eat fewer carbohydrates than when you eat fewer fats. Your weight loss will however plateau faster on a low-carbohydrate diet than on a low-fat diet. This is because these diets cause weight loss through different mechanisms in your body. With the plateau-proof diet, you will alternate between a low-carbohydrate diet and a low-fat diet to prevent the weight loss plateau.

<u>Getting started</u>
To simplify your weight loss process, I highly recommend that you keep a well-organized log until you attain complete weight loss. Start by drawing this chart below in your log, then go back

to Chapter 2 and complete the table. When you complete the table, go to the market and buy the spices that you selected. Immediately make oil infusions (see Chapter 2) of the spices when you return from the market. You should preferably use olive oil to make your infusions, but you can also use other monounsaturated and polyunsaturated oils such as canola oil, peanut oil, cottonseed oil, corn oil, safflower oil, soybean oil, etc. Please note that herbs and spices with the same therapeutic effect typically work through different mechanisms, so combine as many as possible in your infusions.

Desired therapeutic effect (e.g. weight loss or lower blood glucose levels)	My choice of herbs and/or spices (Choose as many as possible)	Type of infusion oil
(1)		
(2)		
(3)		

Once you have drawn the table on the previous page in your weight management log, carefully go through the herbs and spices listed in Chapter 2 and fill in the table. The first infusion should be for weight loss. You can also include herbs and spices that lower blood glucose and blood triglyceride levels in the weight loss infusion, since these herbs and spices also affect weight loss indirectly. Create additional infusions for health conditions that concern you, if necessary. Also, make infusions for conditions that you would like to prevent, e.g. heart disease and cancer.

Clear the cabinets and the refrigerator
Before you go to the market for your herbs and spices, you should clear your kitchen cabinets and refrigerator of all foods that are not compliant with the plateau-proof diet (Chapter 4) or the plateau-proof diet cardio (Chapter 5) – depending on which diet you have chosen. When you restock your cabinets and your refrigerator, you should consider separating the CP rotation foods from the FP rotation foods. This will save you time in the long run.

Donating the foods, that you cleared from your kitchen, to a local food program, is a great way to start your new life, isn't it? I think so, and I hope we are singular in thought.

Copy the table below in your weight management log and fill it in using the plateau-proof diet (plateau-proof diet cardio) green and yellow tables. This is your menu for the week. Try to follow it as strictly as you can. If your lifestyle permits it, split lunch and dinner into two smaller meals – that is, you will eat five meals per day instead of three. If you typically snack between meals, then make a menu table for your snacks as well.

Day	Breakfast	Lunch	Dinner
Monday			
Tuesday			
Wednesday			
Thursday			
Friday			

Now you have your medicinal foods and the plateau-proof diet ready to go. This brings the question – what are you going to drink?

Drinks – where the battle is won or lost

<u>The facts</u>
- Drinking moderate amounts of alcohol (especially red wine) may improve your cardiovascular health and help facilitate your weight loss. Moderate drinking consists of drinking 1-2 drinks per day for 3 or 4 days per week. Each drink consists of about 1.5 ounces of liquor, 5 ounces of wine, or 12 ounces of beer.
- Soft drinks (including many fruit juices) will adversely affect your weight loss, perhaps completely compromising it.
- Sports drinks will adversely affect your health and your weight loss due to their high sodium content.
- Water is good.
- Tea (green and black) is good.
- Dark cocoa is good (no diary, no sugar).
- My herbal tea (Chapter 2) is great for weight loss. If you replace soft drinks with it, you will enjoy a rapid weight loss.

<u>So, what do you drink?</u>
Avoid soft drinks and fruit juices that are not compliant with the plateau-proof diet (plateau-proof diet cardio). Avoid sports drinks. If you currently drink alcohol, continue to due so in moderation (as advised by your doctor). Alcohol consumption should be compliant with the rotations of the plateau-proof diet (plateau-proof diet cardio). Drink water, tea and dark cocoa. For the maximum weight loss boost, drink my herbal weight loss tea. If you need to sweeten your tea or cocoa, please use sugar-free sweeteners (especially during the CP rotation).

You are now ready to go to the market. Have fun shopping!

When it comes to your muscles, a little stimulation goes a long way

<u>The facts</u>
- You may not need any exercise to lose weight on the clinique science weight loss program.
- You will however need very moderate exercise (see Introduction) if your health screen showed higher than normal levels glucose or triglycerides (fat). Very moderate exercise will help your muscles use glucose and fat more efficiently, facilitating your weight loss.
- Too much exercising may adversely affect your weight loss. It is important that you allow adequate time between exercises for your body to recuperate. During this (recuperation) time, your muscles will make the vital changes that will lead to a more efficient burning of glucose and fat.
- You don't benefit from exercise by burning stored calories through physical activity – please don't attempt vigorous exercise as a means of increasing your rate of weight loss.

Why the head wears the crown

We are usually not aware that our brains constantly gather information about us and around us, and then instruct our bodies (subconsciously) to make the appropriate functional and structural changes. Your brain communicates with every cell in your body, including your muscle cells and fat cells, by triggering the release of chemical messengers called hormones. For example, insulin is a hormone that when secreted will cause your muscle cells and other cells of your body to increase the burn rate of glucose and fat.

You can consciously feed information to your brain and have your brain transform the information into instructions for the cells of your body. In the case of weight loss, you can do this by thinking positively. You will need to create a strong mental image of yourself (as you imagine yourself to look after complete weight loss) and actively daydream about this image constantly. The information you are sending to your brain is "I have decided to make this slight rearrangement of my body, so get working on it fast". You are not asking your brain, you are instructing it. It is very important to note that when you instruct your brain, you have to absolutely (100%) believe that it is going to do the work. If you do not believe that your brain will instruct your body to lose weight, your brain will not instruct your body to lose weight. Sending information that you do not believe in to your brain, is the same as trying to deceive your brain – an insurmountable task.

Present your weight loss goals to your brain in a manner that you are most comfortable with: a strong mental image of your skinny self, a smaller size dress or knickers that you attempt to put on each day, a doctored digital image of a thinner version of you on your dresser, etc. Think positively, regardless of whatever failures you have had in the past with weight loss. Talk to your brain often, especially during meals and during exercise – it will listen.

The beginning of the end

By choosing to use the clinique science weight loss system, you have chosen to put your weight problems behind you. Weight loss is typically difficult, which is why I included my herbal weight loss tea in this book – it will give you a big boost. It is also why there are extensive technical discussions in this book. I believe that the more you know about weight loss, the easier it will be for you to lose weight. I hope you will also take a minute to teach others who could use this knowledge. Have a wonderful time with your slimmer look.

Appendix: Your health screening results

Date_____

Screen	Your levels	Desirable levels
Total cholesterol		under 200 mg/dl
HDL cholesterol		45 mg/dl or higher
LDL cholesterol		100 mg/dl or lower
Triglycerides		under 150 mg/dl
Glucose		70-99 mg/dl fasting and below 140 mg/dl non-fasting
Blood pressure		systolic under 120 diastolic under 80
Body Mass Index (BMI)		between 18.5 and 25

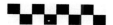

Date_____

Screen	Your levels	Desirable levels
Total cholesterol		under 200 mg/dl
HDL cholesterol		45 mg/dl or higher
LDL cholesterol		100 mg/dl or lower
Triglycerides		under 150 mg/dl
Glucose		70-99 mg/dl fasting and below 140 mg/dl non-fasting
Blood pressure		systolic under 120 diastolic under 80
Body Mass Index (BMI)		between 18.5 and 25

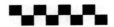

Date_____

Screen	Your levels	Desirable levels
Total cholesterol		under 200 mg/dl
HDL cholesterol		45 mg/dl or higher
LDL cholesterol		100 mg/dl or lower
Triglycerides		under 150 mg/dl
Glucose		70-99 mg/dl fasting and below 140 mg/dl non-fasting
Blood pressure		systolic under 120 diastolic under 80
Body Mass Index (BMI)		between 18.5 and 25

Date_____

Screen	Your levels	Desirable levels
Total cholesterol		under 200 mg/dl
HDL cholesterol		45 mg/dl or higher
LDL cholesterol		100 mg/dl or lower
Triglycerides		under 150 mg/dl
Glucose		70-99 mg/dl fasting and below 140 mg/dl non-fasting
Blood pressure		systolic under 120 diastolic under 80
Body Mass Index (BMI)		between 18.5 and 25

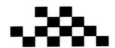

Date_____

Screen	Your levels	Desirable levels
Total cholesterol		under 200 mg/dl
HDL cholesterol		45 mg/dl or higher
LDL cholesterol		100 mg/dl or lower
Triglycerides		under 150 mg/dl
Glucose		70-99 mg/dl fasting and below 140 mg/dl non-fasting
Blood pressure		systolic under 120 diastolic under 80
Body Mass Index (BMI)		between 18.5 and 25

49.   Sanchez-Moreno, C. et al. Consumption of high-pressurized vegetable soup increases plasma vitamin C and decreases oxidative stress and inflammatory biomarkers in healthy humans. *J Nutr* **134**, 3021-5 (2004).

50.   Appel, L.J. et al. A clinical trial of the effects of dietary patterns on blood pressure. DASH Collaborative Research Group. *N Engl J Med* **336**, 1117-24 (1997).

51.   Wertz, K. et al. Beta-carotene inhibits UVA-induced matrix metalloprotease 1 and 10 expression in keratinocytes by a singlet oxygen-dependent mechanism. *Free Radic Biol Med* **37**, 654-70 (2004).

52.   Stahl, W. & Sies, H. Bioactivity and protective effects of natural carotenoids. *Biochim Biophys Acta* **1740**, 101-7 (2005).

53.   Bando, N. et al. Participation of singlet oxygen in ultraviolet-a-induced lipid peroxidation in mouse skin and its inhibition by dietary beta-carotene: an ex vivo study. *Free Radic Biol Med* **37**, 1854-63 (2004).

54.   Cho, E. et al. Red meat intake and risk of breast cancer among premenopausal women. *Arch Intern Med* **166**, 2253-9 (2006).

55.   Gray, G.E., Pike, M.C. & Henderson, B.E. Breast-cancer incidence and mortality rates in different countries in relation to known risk factors and dietary practices. *Br J Cancer* **39**, 1-7 (1979).

56.   Holmes, M.D. et al. Meat, fish and egg intake and risk of breast cancer. *Int J Cancer* **104**, 221-7 (2003).

57.   van der Hel, O.L. et al. GSTM1 null genotype, red meat consumption and breast cancer risk (The Netherlands). *Cancer Causes Control* **15**, 295-303 (2004).

58.   Dai, Q. et al. Consumption of animal foods, cooking methods, and risk of breast cancer. *Cancer Epidemiol Biomarkers Prev* **11**, 801-8 (2002).

59.   Cho, E. et al. Premenopausal fat intake and risk of breast cancer. *J Natl Cancer Inst* **95**, 1079-85 (2003).

60.   Liu, K.H. et al. Sonographic measurement of mesenteric fat thickness is a good correlate with cardiovascular risk factors: comparison with subcutaneous and preperitoneal fat thickness, magnetic resonance imaging and anthropometric indexes. *Int J Obes Relat Metab Disord* **27**, 1267-73 (2003).

61. Goldstone, A.P. et al. Visceral adipose tissue and metabolic complications of obesity are reduced in Prader-Willi syndrome female adults: evidence for novel influences on body fat distribution. *J Clin Endocrinol Metab* **86**, 4330-8 (2001).

62. Pare, A. et al. Is the relationship between adipose tissue and waist girth altered by weight loss in obese men? *Obes Res* **9**, 526-34 (2001).

63. Shojaee-Moradie, F. et al. Exercise training reduces fatty acid availability and improves the insulin sensitivity of glucose metabolism. *Diabetologia* (2006).

64. Barnard, N.D., Scialli, A.R., Turner-McGrievy, G., Lanou, A.J. & Glass, J. The effects of a low-fat, plant-based dietary intervention on body weight, metabolism, and insulin sensitivity. *Am J Med* **118**, 991-7 (2005).

65. Burke, L.E. et al. PREFER study: a randomized clinical trial testing treatment preference and two dietary options in behavioral weight management--rationale, design and baseline characteristics. *Contemp Clin Trials* **27**, 34-48 (2006).

66. Smith, C.F., Burke, L.E. & Wing, R.R. Vegetarian and weight-loss diets among young adults. *Obes Res* **8**, 123-9 (2000).

67. Jenkins, D.J. et al. Type 2 diabetes and the vegetarian diet. *Am J Clin Nutr* **78**, 610S-616S (2003).

68. Nicholson, A.S. et al. Toward improved management of NIDDM: A randomized, controlled, pilot intervention using a lowfat, vegetarian diet. *Prev Med* **29**, 87-91 (1999).

69. Baker, G., Fraser, R.J. & Young, G. Subtypes of functional dyspepsia. *World J Gastroenterol* **12**, 2667-71 (2006).

70. de Souza Pereira, R. Regression of an esophageal ulcer using a dietary supplement containing melatonin. *J Pineal Res* **40**, 355-6 (2006).

71. Yuan, Y., Padol, I.T. & Hunt, R.H. Peptic ulcer disease today. *Nat Clin Pract Gastroenterol Hepatol* **3**, 80-9 (2006).

72. Matysiak-Budnik, T. & Megraud, F. Helicobacter pylori infection and gastric cancer. *Eur J Cancer* **42**, 708-16 (2006).

73. Aro, P. et al. Body mass index and chronic unexplained gastrointestinal symptoms: an adult endoscopic population based study. *Gut* **54**, 1377-83 (2005).

74. Popkin, B.M. et al. A new proposed guidance system for beverage consumption in the United States. *Am J Clin Nutr* **83**, 529-42 (2006).

75. James, J., Thomas, P., Cavan, D. & Kerr, D. Preventing childhood obesity by reducing consumption of carbonated drinks: cluster randomised controlled trial. *Bmj* **328**, 1237 (2004).

76. Striegel-Moore, R.H. et al. Correlates of beverage intake in adolescent girls: the National Heart, Lung, and Blood Institute Growth and Health Study. *J Pediatr* **148**, 183-7 (2006).

77. Murray, R., Frankowski, B. & Taras, H. Are soft drinks a scapegoat for childhood obesity? *J Pediatr* **146**, 586-90 (2005).

78. Raben, A., Vasilaras, T.H., Moller, A.C. & Astrup, A. Sucrose compared with artificial sweeteners: different effects on ad libitum food intake and body weight after 10 wk of supplementation in overweight subjects. *Am J Clin Nutr* **76**, 721-9 (2002).

79. Schulze, M.B. et al. Sugar-sweetened beverages, weight gain, and incidence of type 2 diabetes in young and middle-aged women. *Jama* **292**, 927-34 (2004).

80. Zemel, M.B. et al. Dairy augmentation of total and central fat loss in obese subjects. *Int J Obes (Lond)* **29**, 391-7 (2005).

81. Zemel, M.B. & Miller, S.L. Dietary calcium and dairy modulation of adiposity and obesity risk. *Nutr Rev* **62**, 125-31 (2004).

82. Novotny, R., Daida, Y.G., Acharya, S., Grove, J.S. & Vogt, T.M. Dairy intake is associated with lower body fat and soda intake with greater weight in adolescent girls. *J Nutr* **134**, 1905-9 (2004).

83. Berkey, C.S., Rockett, H.R., Willett, W.C. & Colditz, G.A. Milk, dairy fat, dietary calcium, and weight gain: a longitudinal study of adolescents. *Arch Pediatr Adolesc Med* **159**, 543-50 (2005).

84. Nunn, J.F. Ancient Egyptian medicine. *Trans Med Soc Lond* **113**, 57-68 (1996).

85. Rivlin, R.S. Is garlic alternative medicine? *J Nutr* **136**, 713S-715S (2006).

86. Rahman, K. & Lowe, G.M. Garlic and cardiovascular disease: a critical review. *J Nutr* **136**, 736S-740S (2006).

87. Fleischauer, A.T. & Arab, L. Garlic and cancer: a critical review of the epidemiologic literature. *J Nutr* **131**, 1032S-40S (2001).

88. Borek, C. Garlic reduces dementia and heart-disease risk. *J Nutr* **136**, 810S-812S (2006).

89. Amagase, H. Clarifying the real bioactive constituents of garlic. *J Nutr* **136**, 716S-725S (2006).

90. Watanabe, T., Kawada, T., Kurosawa, M., Sato, A. & Iwai, K. Adrenal sympathetic efferent nerve and catecholamine secretion excitation caused by capsaicin in rats. *Am J Physiol* **255**, E23-7 (1988).

91. Yoshioka, M. et al. Maximum tolerable dose of red pepper decreases fat intake independently of spicy sensation in the mouth. *Br J Nutr* **91**, 991-5 (2004).

92. Yoshioka, M. et al. Effects of red pepper on appetite and energy intake. *Br J Nutr* **82**, 115-23 (1999).

93. Lim, K. et al. Dietary red pepper ingestion increases carbohydrate oxidation at rest and during exercise in runners. *Med Sci Sports Exerc* **29**, 355-61 (1997).

94. Chaiyata, P., Puttadechakum, S. & Komindr, S. Effect of chili pepper (Capsicum frutescens) ingestion on plasma glucose response and metabolic rate in Thai women. *J Med Assoc Thai* **86**, 854-60 (2003).

95. Tolan, I., Ragoobirsingh, D. & Morrison, E.Y. The effect of capsaicin on blood glucose, plasma insulin levels and insulin binding in dog models. *Phytother Res* **15**, 391-4 (2001).

96. Cichewicz, R.H. & Thorpe, P.A. The antimicrobial properties of chile peppers (Capsicum species) and their uses in Mayan medicine. *J Ethnopharmacol* **52**, 61-70 (1996).

97. Steinberg, F.M., Bearden, M.M. & Keen, C.L. Cocoa and chocolate flavonoids: implications for cardiovascular health. *J Am Diet Assoc* **103**, 215-23 (2003).

98. Fisher, N.D. & Hollenberg, N.K. Flavanols for cardiovascular health: the science behind the sweetness. *J Hypertens* **23**, 1453-9 (2005).

99. Keen, C.L., Holt, R.R., Oteiza, P.I., Fraga, C.G. & Schmitz, H.H. Cocoa antioxidants and cardiovascular health. *Am J Clin Nutr* **81**, 298S-303S (2005).

100. Ding, E.L., Hutfless, S.M., Ding, X. & Girotra, S. Chocolate and prevention of cardiovascular disease: a systematic review. *Nutr Metab (Lond)* **3**, 2 (2006).

101. Miller, A.L. Epidemiology, etiology, and natural treatment of seasonal affective disorder. *Altern Med Rev* **10**, 5-13 (2005).

102. Davis, C. & Levitan, R.D. Seasonality and seasonal affective disorder (SAD): an evolutionary viewpoint tied to energy conservation and reproductive cycles. *J Affect Disord* **87**, 3-10 (2005).

103. Barnes, J., Anderson, L.A. & Phillipson, J.D. St John's wort (Hypericum perforatum L.): a review of its chemistry, pharmacology and clinical properties. *J Pharm Pharmacol* **53**, 583-600 (2001).

104. Pouwer, F. et al. Fat food for a bad mood. Could we treat and prevent depression in Type 2 diabetes by means of omega-3 polyunsaturated fatty acids? A review of the evidence. *Diabet Med* **22**, 1465-75 (2005).

105. Paul, R.T., McDonnell, A.P. & Kelly, C.B. Folic acid: neurochemistry, metabolism and relationship to depression. *Hum Psychopharmacol* **19**, 477-88 (2004).

106. Tajuddin, Ahmad, S., Latif, A. & Qasmi, I.A. Aphrodisiac activity of 50% ethanolic extracts of Myristica fragrans Houtt. (nutmeg) and Syzygium aromaticum (L) Merr. & Perry. (clove) in male mice: a comparative study. *BMC Complement Altern Med* **3**, 6 (2003).

107. Tajuddin, Ahmad, S., Latif, A., Qasmi, I.A. & Amin, K.M. An experimental study of sexual function improving effect of Myristica fragrans Houtt. (nutmeg). *BMC Complement Altern Med* **5**, 16 (2005).

108. Sjoholm, A., Lindberg, A. & Personne, M. [A case report. Poisoned by nutmeg]. *Lakartidningen* **94**, 731-2 (1997).

109. Goncalves, J.L. et al. In vitro anti-rotavirus activity of some medicinal plants used in Brazil against diarrhea. *J Ethnopharmacol* **99**, 403-7 (2005).

110. Ram, A., Lauria, P., Gupta, R. & Sharma, V.N. Hypolipidaemic effect of Myristica fragrans fruit extract in rabbits. *J Ethnopharmacol* **55**, 49-53 (1996).

111. van Dam, R.M. & Hu, F.B. Coffee consumption and risk of type 2 diabetes: a systematic review. *Jama* **294**, 97-104 (2005).

112. Westerterp-Plantenga, M.S., Lejeune, M.P. & Kovacs, E.M. Body weight loss and weight maintenance in relation to habitual caffeine intake and green tea supplementation. *Obes Res* **13**, 1195-204 (2005).

113. Astrup, A. et al. Caffeine: a double-blind, placebo-controlled study of its thermogenic, metabolic, and cardiovascular effects in healthy volunteers. *Am J Clin Nutr* **51**, 759-67 (1990).

114. Astrup, A. Thermogenic drugs as a strategy for treatment of obesity. *Endocrine* **13**, 207-12 (2000).

115. Hasegawa, N. Inhibition of lipogenesis by pycnogenol. *Phytother Res* **14**, 472-3 (2000).

116. Bracco, D., Ferrarra, J.M., Arnaud, M.J., Jequier, E. & Schutz, Y. Effects of caffeine on energy metabolism, heart rate, and methylxanthine metabolism in lean and obese women. *Am J Physiol* **269**, E671-8 (1995).

117. Salazar-Martinez, E. et al. Coffee consumption and risk for type 2 diabetes mellitus. *Ann Intern Med* **140**, 1-8 (2004).

118. Nawrot, P. et al. Effects of caffeine on human health. *Food Addit Contam* **20**, 1-30 (2003).

119. Bell, S. et al. Effect of beta-glucan from oats and yeast on serum lipids. *Crit Rev Food Sci Nutr* **39**, 189-202 (1999).

120. Truswell, A.S. Cereal grains and coronary heart disease. *Eur J Clin Nutr* **56**, 1-14 (2002).

121. Ashfield-Watt, P.A., Moat, S.J., Doshi, S.N. & McDowell, I.F. Folate, homocysteine, endothelial function and cardiovascular disease. What is the link? *Biomed Pharmacother* **55**, 425-33 (2001).

122. Erkkila, A.T. & Lichtenstein, A.H. Fiber and Cardiovascular Disease Risk: How Strong Is the Evidence? *J Cardiovasc Nurs* **21**, 3-8 (2006).

123. Anderson, J.W. Whole grains and coronary heart disease: the whole kernel of truth. *Am J Clin Nutr* **80**, 1459-60 (2004).

124. Liu, S. Whole-grain foods, dietary fiber, and type 2 diabetes: searching for a kernel of truth. *Am J Clin Nutr* **77**, 527-9 (2003).

125. Chitturi, S. & George, J. Hepatotoxicity of commonly used drugs: nonsteroidal anti-inflammatory drugs, antihypertensives, antidiabetic agents, anticonvulsants, lipid-lowering agents, psychotropic drugs. *Semin Liver Dis* **22**, 169-83 (2002).

126. Broadhurst, C.L., Polansky, M.M. & Anderson, R.A. Insulin-like biological activity of culinary and medicinal plant aqueous extracts in vitro. *J Agric Food Chem* **48**, 849-52 (2000).

127. Verspohl, E.J., Bauer, K. & Neddermann, E. Antidiabetic effect of Cinnamomum cassia and Cinnamomum zeylanicum in vivo and in vitro. *Phytother Res* **19**, 203-6 (2005).

128. Khan, A., Safdar, M., Ali Khan, M.M., Khattak, K.N. & Anderson, R.A. Cinnamon improves glucose and lipids of people with type 2 diabetes. *Diabetes Care* **26**, 3215-8 (2003).

129. Anderson, R.A. et al. Isolation and characterization of polyphenol type-A polymers from cinnamon with insulin-like biological activity. *J Agric Food Chem* **52**, 65-70 (2004).

130. Kamath, J.V., Rana, A.C. & Chowdhury, A.R. Pro-healing effect of Cinnamomum zeylanicum bark. *Phytother Res* **17**, 970-2 (2003).

131. Qin, B. et al. Cinnamon extract (traditional herb) potentiates in vivo insulin-regulated glucose utilization via enhancing insulin signaling in rats. *Diabetes Res Clin Pract* **62**, 139-48 (2003).

132. Ryttig, K.R., Flaten, H. & Rossner, S. Long-term effects of a very low calorie diet (Nutrilett) in obesity treatment. A prospective, randomized, comparison between VLCD and a hypocaloric diet+behavior modification and their combination. *Int J Obes Relat Metab Disord* **21**, 574-9 (1997).

133. Blanch Miro, S., Recasens Gracia, M.A., Sola Alberich, R. & Salas-Salvado, J. [Effect of a highly hypocaloric diet on the control of morbid obesity in the short and the long term]. *Med Clin (Barc)* **100**, 450-3 (1993).

134. Coleman, M.D. & Nickols-Richardson, S.M. Urinary ketones reflect serum ketone concentration but do not relate to weight loss in overweight premenopausal women following a low-carbohydrate/high-protein diet. *J Am Diet Assoc* **105**, 608-11 (2005).

135. Foster, G.D. et al. A randomized trial of a low-carbohydrate diet for obesity. *N Engl J Med* **348**, 2082-90 (2003).

136. Meckling, K.A., O'Sullivan, C. & Saari, D. Comparison of a low-fat diet to a low-carbohydrate diet on weight loss, body composition, and risk factors for diabetes and cardiovascular disease in free-living, overweight men and women. *J Clin Endocrinol Metab* **89**, 2717-23 (2004).

137. Meckling, K.A., Gauthier, M., Grubb, R. & Sanford, J. Effects of a hypocaloric, low-carbohydrate diet on weight loss, blood lipids, blood pressure, glucose tolerance, and body composition in free-living overweight women. *Can J Physiol Pharmacol* **80**, 1095-105 (2002).

138. Samaha, F.F. et al. A low-carbohydrate as compared with a low-fat diet in severe obesity. *N Engl J Med* **348**, 2074-81 (2003).

139. Seshadri, P. et al. A randomized study comparing the effects of a low-carbohydrate diet and a conventional diet on lipoprotein subfractions and C-reactive protein levels in patients with severe obesity. *Am J Med* **117**, 398-405 (2004).

140. Stern, L. et al. The effects of low-carbohydrate versus conventional weight loss diets in severely obese adults: one-year follow-up of a randomized trial. *Ann Intern Med* **140**, 778-85 (2004).

141. Dessein, P.H., Shipton, E.A., Stanwix, A.E., Joffe, B.I. & Ramokgadi, J. Beneficial effects of weight loss associated with moderate calorie/carbohydrate restriction, and increased proportional intake of protein and unsaturated fat on serum urate and lipoprotein levels in gout: a pilot study. *Ann Rheum Dis* **59**, 539-43 (2000).

142. Layman, D.K. et al. A reduced ratio of dietary carbohydrate to protein improves body composition and blood lipid profiles during weight loss in adult women. *J Nutr* **133**, 411-7 (2003).

143. Lean, M.E., Han, T.S., Prvan, T., Richmond, P.R. & Avenell, A. Weight loss with high and low carbohydrate 1200 kcal diets in free living women. *Eur J Clin Nutr* **51**, 243-8 (1997).

144. Miyashita, Y. et al. Beneficial effect of low carbohydrate in low calorie diets on visceral fat reduction in type 2 diabetic patients with obesity. *Diabetes Res Clin Pract* **65**, 235-41 (2004).

145. Hauner, H. [Low-carbohydrate or low-fat diet for weight loss--which is better?]. *MMW Fortschr Med* **146**, 33-5, 37 (2004).

146. Johnston, C.S., Tjonn, S.L. & Swan, P.D. High-protein, low-fat diets are effective for weight loss and favorably alter biomarkers in healthy adults. *J Nutr* **134**, 586-91 (2004).

147. Brinkworth, G.D., Noakes, M., Parker, B., Foster, P. & Clifton, P.M. Long-term effects of advice to consume a high-protein, low-fat diet, rather than a

conventional weight-loss diet, in obese adults with type 2 diabetes: one-year follow-up of a randomised trial. *Diabetologia* **47**, 1677-86 (2004).

148. Bahadori, B. et al. Low-fat, high-carbohydrate (low-glycaemic index) diet induces weight loss and preserves lean body mass in obese healthy subjects: results of a 24-week study. *Diabetes Obes Metab* **7**, 290-3 (2005).

149. Moyad, M.A. Fad diets and obesity--Part IV: Low-carbohydrate vs. low-fat diets. *Urol Nurs* **25**, 67-70 (2005).

150. Noakes, M., Keogh, J.B., Foster, P.R. & Clifton, P.M. Effect of an energy-restricted, high-protein, low-fat diet relative to a conventional high-carbohydrate, low-fat diet on weight loss, body composition, nutritional status, and markers of cardiovascular health in obese women. *Am J Clin Nutr* **81**, 1298-306 (2005).

151. Sharman, M.J. & Volek, J.S. Weight loss leads to reductions in inflammatory biomarkers after a very-low-carbohydrate diet and a low-fat diet in overweight men. *Clin Sci (Lond)* **107**, 365-9 (2004).

152. Volek, J. et al. Comparison of energy-restricted very low-carbohydrate and low-fat diets on weight loss and body composition in overweight men and women. *Nutr Metab (Lond)* **1**, 13 (2004).

153. Willi, S.M., Oexmann, M.J., Wright, N.M., Collop, N.A. & Key, L.L., Jr. The effects of a high-protein, low-fat, ketogenic diet on adolescents with morbid obesity: body composition, blood chemistries, and sleep abnormalities. *Pediatrics* **101**, 61-7 (1998).

154. Yancy, W.S., Jr., Olsen, M.K., Guyton, J.R., Bakst, R.P. & Westman, E.C. A low-carbohydrate, ketogenic diet versus a low-fat diet to treat obesity and hyperlipidemia: a randomized, controlled trial. *Ann Intern Med* **140**, 769-77 (2004).

155. Benoit, F.L., Martin, R.L. & Watten, R.H. Changes in body composition during weight reduction in obesity. Balance studies comparing effects of fasting and a ketogenic diet. *Ann Intern Med* **63**, 604-12 (1965).

156. Vazquez, J.A. & Adibi, S.A. Protein sparing during treatment of obesity: ketogenic versus nonketogenic very low calorie diet. *Metabolism* **41**, 406-14 (1992).

157. Van Itallie, T.B. Dietary fiber and obesity. *Am J Clin Nutr* **31**, S43-52 (1978).

158. Ullrich, I.H. & Albrink, M.J. The effect of dietary fiber and other factors on insulin response: role in obesity. *J Environ Pathol Toxicol Oncol* **5**, 137-55 (1985).

159. Trallero Casanas, R. [Fiber in the treatment of obesity and its comorbidities]. *Nutr Hosp* **17 Suppl 1**, 17-22 (2002).

160. Southgate, D.A. Has dietary fibre a role in the prevention and treatment of obesity. *Bibl Nutr Dieta*, 70-6 (1978).

161. Smith, U. Dietary fibre, diabetes and obesity. *Int J Obes* **11 Suppl 1**, 27-31 (1987).

162. Silman, A.J. Cereal fibre, total energy intake, and obesity. *Lancet* **2**, 905 (1979).

163. Leeds, A.R. Treatment of obesity with dietary fibre: present position and potential developments. *Scand J Gastroenterol Suppl* **129**, 156-8 (1987).

164. Kimm, S.Y. The role of dietary fiber in the development and treatment of childhood obesity. *Pediatrics* **96**, 1010-4 (1995).

165. Kaul, L. & Nidiry, J. High-fiber diet in the treatment of obesity and hypercholesterolemia. *J Natl Med Assoc* **85**, 231-2 (1993).

166. Gropper, S.S. & Acosta, P.B. The therapeutic effect of fiber in treating obesity. *J Am Coll Nutr* **6**, 533-5 (1987).

167. Baron, J.A., Schori, A., Crow, B., Carter, R. & Mann, J.I. A randomized controlled trial of low carbohydrate and low fat/high fiber diets for weight loss. *Am J Public Health* **76**, 1293-6 (1986).

168. Andersson, B., Terning, K. & Bjorntorp, P. Dietary treatment of obesity localized in different regions. The effect of dietary fibre on relapse. *Int J Obes* **11 Suppl 1**, 79-85 (1987).

169. Anderson, J.W. & Bryant, C.A. Dietary fiber: diabetes and obesity. *Am J Gastroenterol* **81**, 898-906 (1986).

170. Albrink, M.J. Dietary fiber, plasma insulin, and obesity. *Am J Clin Nutr* **31**, S277-S279 (1978).

171. Kritchevsky, D. & Story, J.A. Dietary fiber and cancer. *Curr Concepts Nutr* **6**, 41-54 (1977).

172. Burkitt, D.P. Colonic-rectal cancer: fiber and other dietary factors. *Am J Clin Nutr* **31**, S58-S64 (1978).

173. Esser, W., Weithofer, G. & Bloch, R. [The significance of dietary fat and fiber for the aetiology of colon cancer (author's transl)]. *Z Gastroenterol* **18**, 30-7 (1980).

174. Talbot, J.M. Role of dietary fiber in diverticular disease and colon cancer. *Fed Proc* **40**, 2337-42 (1981).

175. Kritchevsky, D. Dietary fiber and cancer. *Nutr Cancer* **6**, 213-9 (1984).

176. Bright-See, E. et al. Dietary fiber and cancer: a supplement for intervention studies. *Nutr Cancer* **7**, 211-20 (1985).

177. Greenwald, P. & Lanza, E. Role of dietary fiber in the prevention of cancer. *Important Adv Oncol*, 37-54 (1986).

178. Klurfeld, D.M. & Kritchevsky, D. Dietary fiber and human cancer: critique of the literature. *Adv Exp Med Biol* **206**, 119-35 (1986).

179. Jacobs, L.R. Relationship between dietary fiber and cancer: metabolic, physiologic, and cellular mechanisms. *Proc Soc Exp Biol Med* **183**, 299-310 (1986).

180. Ho, E.E., Atwood, J.R. & Meyskens, F.L., Jr. Methodological development of dietary fiber intervention to lower colon cancer risk. *Prog Clin Biol Res* **248**, 263-81 (1987).

181. Burkitt, D.P. Dietary fiber and cancer. *J Nutr* **118**, 531-3 (1988).

182. Rose, D.P. Dietary fiber and breast cancer. *Nutr Cancer* **13**, 1-8 (1990).

183. Cheah, P.Y. & Bernstein, H. Colon cancer and dietary fiber: cellulose inhibits the DNA-damaging ability of bile acids. *Nutr Cancer* **13**, 51-7 (1990).

184. Ross, J.K., Pusateri, D.J. & Shultz, T.D. Dietary and hormonal evaluation of men at different risks for prostate cancer: fiber intake, excretion, and composition, with in vitro evidence for an association between steroid hormones and specific fiber components. *Am J Clin Nutr* **51**, 365-70 (1990).

185. Fuchs, C.S. et al. Dietary fiber and the risk of colorectal cancer and adenoma in women. *N Engl J Med* **340**, 169-76 (1999).

186. Reddy, B.S. Role of dietary fiber in colon cancer: an overview. *Am J Med* **106**, 16S-19S; discussion 50S-51S (1999).

187. Honda, T., Kai, I. & Ohi, G. Fat and dietary fiber intake and colon cancer mortality: a chronological comparison between Japan and the United States. *Nutr Cancer* **33**, 95-9 (1999).

188. Terry, P., Jain, M., Miller, A.B., Howe, G.R. & Rohan, T.E. No association among total dietary fiber, fiber fractions, and risk of breast cancer. *Cancer Epidemiol Biomarkers Prev* **11**, 1507-8 (2002).

189. Protein-sparing diets. *Med Lett Drugs Ther* **19**, 69-70 (1977).

190. "Liquid protein diets" and "protein-sparing modified fast". *N Engl J Med* **299**, 419-21 (1978).

191. Use of protein-sparing modified fast in treatment of diabetes and obesity. *J Tenn Med Assoc* **72**, 682-4 (1979).

192. Bell, L., Chan, L. & Pencharz, P.B. Protein-sparing diet for severely obese adolescents: design and use of an equivalency system for menu planning. *J Am Diet Assoc* **85**, 459-64 (1985).

193. Bellows, J.G. & Bellows, R.T. Protein-sparing diet therapy. *Compr Ther* **4**, 3-4 (1978).

194. Bistrian, D.R., Winterer, J., Blackburn, G.L., Young, V. & Sherman, M. Effect of a protein-sparing diet and brief fast on nitrogen metabolism in mildly obese subjects. *J Lab Clin Med* **89**, 1030-5 (1977).

195. Bistrian, B.R., Blackburn, G.L. & Stanbury, J.B. Metabolic aspects of a protein-sparing modified fast in the dietary management of Prader-Willi obesity. *N Engl J Med* **296**, 774-9 (1977).

196. Bistrian, B.R. Clinical use of a protein-sparing modified fast. *Jama* **240**, 2299-302 (1978).

197. Bistrian, B.R. & Sherman, M. Results of the treatment of obesity with a protein-sparing modified fast. *Int J Obes* **2**, 143-8 (1978).

198. Contaldo, F., Di Biase, G., Scalfi, L., Presta, E. & Mancini, M. Protein-sparing modified fast in the treatment of severe obesity: weight loss and nitrogen balance data. *Int J Obes* **4**, 189-96 (1980).

199. Craig, D.W. Treatment of morbid obesity with protein-sparing modified fast. *J Ark Med Soc* **78**, 489-96 (1982).

200. Everse, J.W. Recent developments in protein-sparing therapy. *Hormoner* **12**, 1-14 (1959).

201. Iselin, H.U. & Burckhardt, P. Balanced hypocaloric diet versus protein-sparing modified fast in the treatment of obesity: a comparative study. *Int J Obes* **6**, 175-81 (1982).

202. Jourdan, M., Margen, S. & Bradfield, R.B. Protein-sparing effect in obese women fed low calorie diets. *Am J Clin Nutr* **27**, 3-12 (1974).

203. Seim, H.C. & Rigden, S.R. Approaching the protein-sparing modified fast. *Am Fam Physician* **42**, 51S-56S (1990).

204. Vermeulen, A. Effects of a short-term (4 weeks) protein-sparing modified fast on plasma lipids and lipoproteins in obese women. *Ann Nutr Metab* **34**, 133-42 (1990).

205. Wadden, T.A., Stunkard, A.J., Brownell, K.D. & Day, S.C. A comparison of two very-low-calorie diets: protein-sparing-modified fast versus protein-formula-liquid diet. *Am J Clin Nutr* **41**, 533-9 (1985).

206. Brown, J.M., Yetter, J.F., Spicer, M.J. & Jones, J.D. Cardiac complications of protein-sparing modified fasting. *Jama* **240**, 120-2 (1978).

207. Ebbeling, C.B., Leidig, M.M., Sinclair, K.B., Hangen, J.P. & Ludwig, D.S. A reduced-glycemic load diet in the treatment of adolescent obesity. *Arch Pediatr Adolesc Med* **157**, 773-9 (2003).

208. Banting, W. *Letter on corpulence : addressed to the public*, 22 p. (Printed by Harrison and Sons, [London], 1863).

209. Blanchard, G. et al. Rapid weight loss with a high-protein low-energy diet allows the recovery of ideal body composition and insulin sensitivity in obese dogs. *J Nutr* **134**, 2148S-2150S (2004).

210. Donini, L.M., Pinto, A. & Cannella, C. [High-protein diets and obesity]. *Ann Ital Med Int* **19**, 36-42 (2004).

211. Eisenstein, J., Roberts, S.B., Dallal, G. & Saltzman, E. High-protein weight-loss diets: are they safe and do they work? A review of the experimental and epidemiologic data. *Nutr Rev* **60**, 189-200 (2002).

212. Fitz, J.D., Sperling, E.M. & Fein, H.G. A hypocaloric high-protein diet as primary therapy for adults with obesity-related diabetes: effective long-term use in a community hospital. *Diabetes Care* **6**, 328-33 (1983).

213. Howard, A.N. & Anderson, T.B. The treatment of obesity with a high-protein loaf. *Practitioner* **201**, 491-6 (1968).

214. Johnston, C.S., Day, C.S. & Swan, P.D. Postprandial thermogenesis is increased 100% on a high-protein, low-fat diet versus a high-carbohydrate, low-fat diet in healthy, young women. *J Am Coll Nutr* **21**, 55-61 (2002).

215. Korobov, D.M. & Petrosian, A.A. [Experience with a high-protein reducing diet in the treatment of obesity]. *Vopr Pitan* **26**, 62-4 (1967).

216. Luscombe, N.D., Clifton, P.M., Noakes, M., Farnsworth, E. & Wittert, G. Effect of a high-protein, energy-restricted diet on weight loss and energy expenditure after weight stabilization in hyperinsulinemic subjects. *Int J Obes Relat Metab Disord* **27**, 582-90 (2003).

217. Parker, B., Noakes, M., Luscombe, N. & Clifton, P. Effect of a high-protein, high-monounsaturated fat weight loss diet on glycemic control and lipid levels in type 2 diabetes. *Diabetes Care* **25**, 425-30 (2002).

218. Robinson, S.M. et al. Protein turnover and thermogenesis in response to high-protein and high-carbohydrate feeding in men. *Am J Clin Nutr* **52**, 72-80 (1990).

219. Worthington, B.S. & Taylor, L.E. Balanced low-calorie vs. high-protein-low-carbohydrate reducing diets. I. Weight loss, nutrient intake, and subjective evaluation. *J Am Diet Assoc* **64**, 47-51 (1974).

220. Bowen, J., Noakes, M. & Clifton, P.M. Effect of calcium and dairy foods in high protein, energy-restricted diets on weight loss and metabolic parameters in overweight adults. *Int J Obes Relat Metab Disord* (2005).

221. Clifton, P.M., Noakes, M., Keogh, J. & Foster, P. Effect of an energy reduced high protein red meat diet on weight loss and metabolic parameters in obese women. *Asia Pac J Clin Nutr* **12 Suppl**, S10 (2003).

222. Garcia de los Rios, M., Carrasco, E., Padilla, M., Fonseca, B. & Lopez, G. [Treatment of obesity with a liquid, relatively high protein diet (author's transl)]. *Rev Med Chil* **108**, 691-6 (1980).

223. Halton, T.L. & Hu, F.B. The effects of high protein diets on thermogenesis, satiety and weight loss: a critical review. *J Am Coll Nutr* **23**, 373-85 (2004).

224. Westerterp-Plantenga, M.S., Rolland, V., Wilson, S.A. & Westerterp, K.R. Satiety related to 24 h diet-induced thermogenesis during high protein/carbohydrate vs high fat diets measured in a respiration chamber. *Eur J Clin Nutr* **53**, 495-502 (1999).

225. Westerterp-Plantenga, M.S., Lejeune, M.P., Nijs, I., van Ooijen, M. & Kovacs, E.M. High protein intake sustains weight maintenance after body weight loss in humans. *Int J Obes Relat Metab Disord* **28**, 57-64 (2004).

226. Zed, C. & James, W.P. Dietary thermogenesis in obesity. Response to carbohydrate and protein meals: the effect of beta-adrenergic blockade and semistarvation. *Int J Obes* **10**, 391-405 (1986).

227. Watanabe, A., Wakabayashi, H. & Kuwabara, Y. Nutrient-induced thermogenesis and protein-sparing effect by rapid infusion of a branched chain-enriched amino acid solution to cirrhotic patients. *J Med* **27**, 176-82 (1996).

228. Soucy, J. & Leblanc, J. Protein meals and postprandial thermogenesis. *Physiol Behav* **65**, 705-9 (1999).

229. Schutz, Y., Bray, G. & Margen, S. Postprandial thermogenesis at rest and during exercise in elderly men ingesting two levels of protein. *J Am Coll Nutr* **6**, 497-506 (1987).

230. Garrow, J.S. The contribution of protein synthesis to thermogenesis in man. *Int J Obes* **9 Suppl 2**, 97-101 (1985).

231. Brito, M.N., Botion, L.M., Brito, N.A., Kettelhut, I.C. & Migliorini, R.H. Lipolysis and glycerokinase activity in brown adipose tissue of rat fed a high protein, carbohydrate-free diet. *Horm Metab Res* **26**, 51-2 (1994).

232. Kettelhut, I.C., Foss, M.C. & Migliorini, R.H. Lipolysis and the antilipolytic effect of insulin in adipocytes from rats adapted to a high-protein diet. *Metabolism* **34**, 69-73 (1985).

233. Megia, A. et al. Protein intake during aggressive calorie restriction in obesity determines growth hormone response to growth hormone-releasing hormone after weight loss. *Clin Endocrinol (Oxf)* **39**, 217-20 (1993).

234. Rasmussen, M.H., Juul, A., Kjems, L.L., Skakkebaek, N.E. & Hilsted, J. Lack of stimulation of 24-hour growth hormone release by hypocaloric diet in obesity. *J Clin Endocrinol Metab* **80**, 796-801 (1995).

235. Tanaka, K. et al. Very-low-calorie diet-induced weight reduction reverses impaired growth hormone secretion response to growth hormone-releasing hormone, arginine, and L-dopa in obesity. *Metabolism* **39**, 892-6 (1990).

236. Hara, M. et al. Effects of a low-protein diet on prolactin- and growth hormone-producing cells in the rat pituitary gland. *Anat Rec* **251**, 37-43 (1998).

237. Heffernan, M.A. et al. Increase of fat oxidation and weight loss in obese mice caused by chronic treatment with human growth hormone or a modified C-terminal fragment. *Int J Obes Relat Metab Disord* **25**, 1442-9 (2001).

238. Rasmussen, M.H. et al. Massive weight loss restores 24-hour growth hormone release profiles and serum insulin-like growth factor-I levels in obese subjects. *J Clin Endocrinol Metab* **80**, 1407-15 (1995).

239. Anderson, I.M., Crook, W.S., Gartside, S.E., Fairburn, C.G. & Cowen, P.J. The effect of moderate weight loss on overnight growth hormone and cortisol secretion in healthy female volunteers. *J Affect Disord* **16**, 197-202 (1989).